M. Sandra Wood

Internet Guide
to Cosmetic Surgery
for Men

Pre-publication
REVIEWS,
COMMENTARIES,
EVALUATIONS . . .

"**W**omen are not the only ones opting for 'extreme makeovers' these days, more men than ever before are choosing to undergo cosmetic surgery. The decision whether or not to have cosmetic surgery is a difficult one. There is so much to consider. How does one find a qualified cosmetic surgeon? What types of procedures are available? What are the possible side effects or contraindications? It is hard to know where to begin. M. Sandra Wood's *Internet Guide to Cosmetic Surgery for Men* is a comprehensive, well-organized, and easy-to-use resource that provides answers to these and many other questions.

Internet Guide to Cosmetic Surgery for Men begins with the very basics, showing the reader how to find quality information on the Internet. After a brief dis-

cussion of how to find a good cosmetic surgeon online, and the intricacies of credentialing and board certification, the main portion of this book covers many cosmetic surgery procedures including hair transplantation, body contouring, surgery of the face, head, neck and skin, and cosmetic dentistry. The chapter on ethnic and minority differences in cosmetic procedures, an often neglected topic, is a welcome addition. Keeping the special needs of male health care consumers in mind, this guide contains an excellent combination of commercial, not-for-profit, and educational Web sites. Special features, such as physician locators, chat rooms, message boards, and photo galleries, are highlighted.

Internet Guide to Cosmetic Surgery for Men is an excellent tool to help men make informed decisions regarding cosmetic surgery."

Nancy R. Glassman, MLS, AHIP
Information Technology Librarian,
D. Samuel Gottesman Library,
Albert Einstein College of Medicine

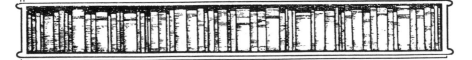

More pre-publication
REVIEWS, COMMENTARIES, EVALUATIONS . . .

"The *Internet Guide to Cosmetic Surgery for Men* provides information on topics related to the location of reliable information on the World Wide Web. This primer on basic Internet searching techniques highlights some excellent sites that are organized by procedure. The book also contains some must-read information on locating a reliable, competent surgeon, while assisting readers to understand credentialing and board certification of clinicians.

This would be an excellent addition to the collection of any public or consumer health library, as well as for the individual who is contemplating a surgical procedure and wants to do some preliminary investigation."

Roberta Bronson Fitzpatrick, MLIS
Associate Director,
UMDNJ–George F. Smith Library
of the Health Sciences

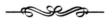

"As cosmetic surgery becomes acceptable and even chic in mainstream society, men as well as women are beginning to consider it as an option to improve their appearance or fight the signs of aging. Since all surgical procedures have risks, anyone thinking about an operation that may radically alter the way they look will want to make sure that they fully understand the procedure. M. Sandra Wood, an experienced medical librarian and the author of a book about cosmetic surgery for women, has written a guide to help men make informed decisions about cosmetic surgical procedures.

Since the Internet has become a major source of medical information, Wood teaches men how to use it. She explains the structure of the World Wide Web, the use of browsers, search engines, and megasites, and basic search strategies. She also shows them how to evaluate the quality of the information about cosmetic surgery. These include sites from professional medical specialty boards, as well as a few sites created by patients who describe their experiences. She covers choosing a physician, general information about surgery, and specific procedures such as liposuction, rhinoplasty, and male breast surgery as well as hair transplantation, cosmetic dentistry, scar and tattoo removal, and Botox injections. Wood even includes information on cosmetic surgeons in other countries. This comprehensive guide to online information about cosmetic surgery is a valuable resource for any man considering a procedure. It belongs in all medical, consumer health, and public libraries."

Barbara M. Bibel, MA, MLS
Consumer Health Information Specialist,
Oakland Public Library,
Oakland, CA

More pre-publication
REVIEWS, COMMENTARIES, EVALUATIONS . . .

"This book will take men from learning the basics about Internet searching, finding quality sites, evaluating those sites, to finding the right surgeon. Along the way they will learn pretty much all they need to know about the procedures and the surgeons. Included are chapters on hair transplantation and cosmetic dentistry to round out the process. Of particular interest are the descriptions of the numerous procedures one might select to undergo, giving the reader and prospective patient full knowledge of what he is getting into. If you are one of those men who has not yet awaken to smell the coffee, cosmetic surgery for men is most definitely in. Why shouldn't men have a little something done to make ourselves look and feel better? This reviewer recently had his eyes done and looks at least ten years younger (or so they tell me). Anyway guys, go for it and this book will be of tremendous help."

Thomas L. Williams, AHIP, MSLS
Professor and Director,
Biomedical Libraries,
University of South Alabama,
College of Medicine

The Haworth Information Press®
An Imprint of The Haworth Press, Inc.
New York • London • Oxford

Internet Guide to Cosmetic Surgery for Men

THE HAWORTH INFORMATION PRESS®
Haworth Internet Medical Guides
M. Sandra Wood, MLS
Editor

The Guide to Complementary and Alternative Medicine on the Internet by Lillian R. Brazin

Internet Guide to Travel Health by Elizabeth Connor

Internet Guide to Food Safety and Security by Elizabeth Connor

Internet Guide to Cosmetic Surgery for Women by M. Sandra Wood

Internet Guide to Anti-Aging and Longevity by Elizabeth Connor

Internet Guide to Herbal Remedies by David J. Owen

Internet Guide to Medical Diets and Nutrition by Lillian R. Brazin

Internet Guide to Cosmetic Surgery for Men by M. Sandra Wood

Internet Guide to Cosmetic Surgery for Men

M. Sandra Wood

The Haworth Information Press®
An Imprint of The Haworth Press, Inc.
New York • London • Oxford

For more information on this book or to order, visit
http://www.haworthpress.com/store/product.asp?sku=5854

or call 1-800-HAWORTH (800-429-6784) in the United States and Canada
or (607) 722-5857 outside the United States and Canada

or contact orders@HaworthPress.com

Published by

The Haworth Information Press®, an imprint of The Haworth Press, Inc., 10 Alice Street, Binghamton, NY
13904-1580.

PUBLISHER'S NOTE
The development, preparation, and publication of this work has been undertaken with great care. However,
the Publisher, employees, editors, and agents of The Haworth Press are not responsible for any errors
contained herein or for consequences that may ensue from use of materials or information contained in this
work. The Haworth Press is committed to the dissemination of ideas and information according to the
highest standards of intellectual freedom and the free exchange of ideas. Statements made and opinions
expressed in this publication do not necessarily reflect the views of the Publisher, Directors, management,
or staff of The Haworth Press, Inc., or an endorsement by them.

Due to the ever-changing nature of the Internet, Web site names and addresses, though verified to the best
of the publisher's ability, should not be accepted as accurate without independent verification.

Cover design by Kerry E. Mack.

Library of Congress Cataloging-in-Publication Data

Wood, M. Sandra.
Internet guide to cosmetic surgery for men / M. Sandra Wood.
p. cm.
Includes bibliographical references and index.
ISBN-13: 978-0-7890-1608-9 (hard : alk. paper)
ISBN-10: 0-7890-1608-7 (hard : alk. paper)
ISBN-13: 978-0-7890-1609-6 (soft : alk. paper)
ISBN-10: 0-7890-1609-5 (soft : alk. paper)
1. Surgery, Plastic—Computer network resources. 2. Men—Surgery—Computer network resources.
3. Internet addresses. 4. Web sites. I. Title.

RD119.W65 2006
617.9′500285—dc22   2006006177

CONTENTS

Abbreviations   ix

Symbol Key   xi

Introduction   1

Chapter 1. Cosmetic Plastic Surgery—The Facts   5

    What Is Plastic Surgery?   6
    Cosmetic Surgery Is a Hot Trend   6
    What Are the Numbers?   8
    How Much Does It Cost?   10
    Why Read This Book?   10

Chapter 2. The Internet—A Brief Look at Where to Begin   13

    The Internet   13
    Internet Addresses   14
    My Site Is Gone!   14
    Evaluating Web Sites: The "Good" versus the "Bad"   15
    Basic Internet Searching   17
    Searching via Your Internet Browser   18
    Searching via a Search Engine/Directory   18
    Searching via a Megasite   21
    Moving on to Specific Sites   24

Chapter 3. Checking Out Credentials   25

    How to Find a Good Cosmetic Surgeon   25
    Credentials/Board Certification   27
    Locating/Selecting a Cosmetic Surgeon Online   33
    Next: Basic Cosmetic Surgery Sites on the Internet   34

Chapter 4. Basic/Core Sites on Cosmetic Surgery   35

    General Sites (.org) on Cosmetic Surgery Procedures   36
    General Sites (.com) on Cosmetic Surgery Procedures   44

General Sites on Cosmetic Surgery for Men   49
Next: Internet Sites for Specific Cosmetic Surgery Procedures   51

Chapter 5. Body Contouring   53

Body Contouring—General   53
Abdominal Liposculpture (Liposuction)   54
Arm Lift (Brachioplasty)/Arm Liposuction/Upper Arm Lift   54
Buttock Augmentation/Implant   57
Buttock Lift/Liposculpture/Liposuction   57
Calf Augmentation/Implants   58
Liposuction   59
Lower Body Lift   67
Thigh Liposuction (Thighplasty)/Thigh Lift   67
Tummy Tuck (Abdominoplasty)   68

Chapter 6. Cosmetic Procedures Specific to Men   73

Gynecomastia-Male Breast Reduction   73
Pectoral (Male Chest) Augmentation/Implants   77
Penis Enlargement/Implants (Phalloplasty)   80

Chapter 7. Cosmetic Surgery of the Face, Head, and Neck   85

Face, Head, and Neck—General   85
Buccal Fat Pad Removal   89
Cheek Implants (Augmentation)   90
Chin Augmentation (Mentoplasty)   91
Ear Surgery (Otoplasty)   94
Eyelid Surgery (Blepharoplasty)   97
Facelift (Rhytidectomy)   100
Facial Implants   103
Facial Liposuction   105
Forehead Lift (Brow Lift)   107
Jaw Augmentation   109
Lip Augmentation   111
Lip Reduction   113
Neck Lift/Neck Liposuction   114
Nose Surgery (Rhinoplasty)   115

Chapter 8. Cosmetic Surgery of the Skin   121

Skin—General   121
Botulinum Toxin (Botox) Injections   124

Cellulite Treatment   128
Chemical Peels   130
Dermabrasion   132
Injectable Fillers   135
Laser Hair Removal   141
Laser Skin Resurfacing   142
Laser Treatment of Spider Veins   145
Microdermabrasion   146
Micropigmentation (Permanent Makeup)   147
Scars/Scar Revision   149
Sclerotherapy   152
Skin Resurfacing   154
Tattoo Removal   156
Thermage   158
Wrinkle Treatment   158

Chapter 9. Hair Transplantation for Men   **161**
Hair Transplantation Sites   163

Chapter 10. Cosmetic Dentistry   **175**
Cosmetic Dentistry Sites   176

Chapter 11. Cosmetic Surgery and Ethnicity   **183**
Ethnic Cosmetic Surgery Sites   184

Chapter 12. International Cosmetic Surgery Associations **187**
International/Multinational Associations   188
Cosmetic Surgery Associations by Country   189

Index   **195**

ABOUT THE AUTHOR

M. Sandra Wood, MLS, MBA, AHIP, FMLA, Librarian Emeritus, University Libraries, The Pennsylvania State University at Hershey. She has more than three decades experience as a medical reference librarian, including the areas of general reference services, management of reference services, database and Internet searching, and user instruction. Ms. Wood has been widely published in the field of medical reference and is editor of *Medical Reference Services Quarterly, Journal of Consumer Health on the Internet,* and *Journal of Electronic Resources in Medical Libraries.* She is editor or co-editor of several books, including *Internet Guide to Cosmetic Surgery for Women, Women's Health on the Internet, Health Care Resources on the Internet: A Guide for Librarians and Health Care Consumers, Men's Health on the Internet,* and *Cancer Resources on the Internet.* She is a member of the Medical Library Association and the Special Libraries Association, and has served on the MLA's Board of Director as Treasurer. Ms. Wood is also a Fellow of the Medical Library Association.

ABBREVIATIONS

AACD	American Academy of Cosmetic Dentistry
AACS	American Academy of Cosmetic Surgery
AAD	American Academy of Dermatology
AAFPRS	American Academy of Facial Plastic and Reconstructive Surgery
ABD	American Board of Dermatology
ABFPRS	American Board of Facial Plastic and Reconstructive Surgery
ABMS	American Board of Medical Specialists
ABO	American Board of Ophthalmology
ABOto	American Board of Otolaryngology
ABPS	American Board of Plastic Surgery
ABS	American Board of Surgery
ASAPS	American Society for Aesthetic Plastic Surgery
ASDS	American Society for Dermatologic Surgery
ASOPRS	American Society of Ophthalmic Plastic and Reconstructive Surgery
ASPS	American Society of Plastic Surgeons
FAQ	frequently asked question
FPSN	Facial Plastic Surgery Network
HON	Health on the Net
html	hypertext markup language
http	hypertext transfer protocol
NOAH	New York Online Access to Health
PDF	portable document format
URL	uniform resource locator

Internet Guide to Cosmetic Surgery for Men
© 2006 by The Haworth Press, Inc. All rights reserved.
doi:10.1300/5854_a

SYMBOL KEY

✎   Blog

📌   Bulletin board

☕   Chat room

🦷   Dentist locator

☀   Discussion forum

✉   Message board

📷   Photo gallery

⚕   Physician locator

⑤   Specialist locator

🤝   Support forum

✚   Technician locator

Internet Guide to Cosmetic Surgery for Men
© 2006 by The Haworth Press, Inc. All rights reserved.
doi:10.1300/5854_b

Introduction

Why write a book about locating information on cosmetic surgery, and why have separate books for men and women? To make a long story short—cosmetic surgery is a "hot" trend that has increased rapidly in popularity. Since it involves permanent changes to your appearance, it follows that you would want to know as much about a procedure as possible before deciding to have cosmetic surgery, and that you would want enough information to make an informed selection of a good surgeon.

In researching information for my first book on this topic, *Internet Guide to Cosmetic Surgery for Women,*[1] I realized that there were enough differences in surgical procedures and special considerations based on sex that two books would be a better approach than a merged book. Yes, there will be major overlaps in sites, but men might not look closely enough at a general cosmetic surgery book that featured Web pages with pictures of women. Statistics show that cosmetic procedures for men represent one of the fastest growing markets in cosmetic surgery. By the time this book is published, I expect that many more sites—both new ones along with special pages on existing sites of some professional association sites—will be directed toward men, as this market is only now beginning to be tapped.

First, though, why my personal interest in cosmetic surgery? I am the original candidate for an "extreme makeover"—the TV show might have been named after me. Tummy tuck, belt lipectomy, liposuction, thigh lipoplasty, breast lift, spider veins, hair replacement, eyelid surgery (both undereye bags and drooping eyelids), wrinkle removal, facial liposuction for double chin—I would be a candidate for all of these procedures and, believe me, have considered all of them over the years and especially while researching and compiling this book and the book for women. Ah, if I just had the money!

My interest in cosmetic surgery began many years ago. As someone who was constantly battling weight, I'd considered having cosmetic surgery but knew that it was not a solution to my problem. Following the birth of my son in 1989, my stomach did not go back to where it had been. Not

Internet Guide to Cosmetic Surgery for Men
© 2006 by The Haworth Press, Inc. All rights reserved.
doi:10.1300/5854_01

that it was ever truly "flat," but after two cesarean sections, the stomach muscles were pretty much gone, and I started thinking about having a tummy tuck. I even got to the point of discussing it with a cosmetic surgeon several years later, following an injury to my forehead which required thirty-one stitches. At a follow-up evaluation to determine whether scar revision would be necessary (it wasn't), I discussed both a tummy tuck and eyelid surgery with the cosmetic surgeon. To this day, I regret my decision not to have the surgery. As part of the baby-boomer generation, I'm not getting any younger, and cosmetic surgery continues to sound attractive.

It used to be that if you had cosmetic surgery, you didn't talk about it. It was something that just happened (e.g., you went away on a "vacation" and came back looking very "rested"). Basically, times have changed since the early to mid-1990s. Perhaps it's the fact that movie stars are talking openly about their cosmetic surgery. Or, possibly it's because every week (sometimes every day), cosmetic surgery is the topic of a TV news or talk show. It's been the focus of several reality shows (e.g., *Extreme Makeover*) and an FX show, *Nip/Tuck*. Or, it may be that the baby-boomer generation, looking to find its youth again—into the "antiaging" frame of mind—has brought cosmetic surgery into the mainstream. Everyday, "real" people, not just movie stars, are talking about cosmetic procedures, from the new "in" procedure, Botox, to the immensely popular surgical procedures of liposuction and hair transplantation. Men are finding that looking younger can have benefits in the job market, from job interviews to promotions. Cosmetic surgery can give you the "one step up" on others seeking the same job.

So, if you are among the increasing number of men considering cosmetic surgery, how do you decide what procedure you want done? How do you find out information about the procedures and treatments that are available and how they are performed? How do you locate a qualified physician? These are the types of questions that this book is intended to help you answer.

The growth of the Internet during the 1990s has opened up ready access to all types of information. It didn't take long before the health care world realized that this was an appropriate way to transmit information to patients and consumers—including information about plastic/cosmetic surgery. The amount of information available on the Internet about cosmetic surgery and various over-the-counter cosmetic therapies is absolutely mind-boggling. Information is available online from professional associations, the government, educational institutions, physicians advertising their private practices, companies selling their products, physician locator services, and more. There is so much to sort through that it becomes difficult and time-consuming to decide which sites to access, let alone which sites are reputable. This book is intended to help you locate quality information about cosmetic surgery on the Internet, guiding you to sites where you can begin your search.

The book is organized into twelve chapters. The first four chapters provide basic information. Chapter 1 introduces plastic and cosmetic surgery, including some definitions, discusses cosmetic surgery as a "hot" trend, and includes statistics on the number of men in the United States having cosmetic surgery. Chapter 2 covers some Internet basics (if you are a beginner with the Internet, you may want to consider purchasing a separate Internet guide). This chapter helps you to evaluate sites, covers basic searching of the Internet, and recommends two megasites for consumer health information. Deciding to have cosmetic surgery involves both the decision of what procedure you want and choosing a physician. Chapter 3 covers physician qualifications, including board certification and membership organizations (and their Web sites), to help you select a physician. Chapter 4 introduces you to basic sites that provide cosmetic surgery information for both men and women. At the end of the chapter are two general sites directed at men. One site is totally devoted to cosmetic surgery in men and scheduled to "go live" while this book is in production. The other site is a special page for cosmetic surgery in men that is part of a professional organization's Web site.

In the next four chapters, cosmetic procedures have been divided into logical groupings: body contouring; cosmetic procedures specific to men; cosmetic surgery of the face, head, and neck; and cosmetic surgery of the skin. Procedures are listed alphabetically under their "common" name, and there are cross-references from the technical names, plus plenty of suggestions to guide you to other related procedures. You will find many of the same sites listed in all chapters, just under different cosmetic procedures.

These chapters are followed by chapters on Web sites for hair transplantation, one of the top procedures for men, and cosmetic dentistry. Chapter 11 discusses ethnic and minority differences in cosmetic procedures. This chapter was added based on comments about the companion book for women. The final chapter lists selected Web sites for professional organizations outside the United States. Cosmetic surgery has been popular outside the United States for many years, and many people travel worldwide to clinics specializing in particular procedures. These organizations provide information that might prove useful should you be considering cosmetic surgery in another country.

One final caution must be noted: These sites are intended as starting points for you to gather information about cosmetic surgery and to locate the physician who might perform your cosmetic procedure. Ultimately, the decision of whether or not to have surgery should be made between you and your physician, and you are encouraged to discuss details of the procedure with him or her. You are urged to check your physician's credentials, including board certification and professional affiliations, and to evaluate previous work that he or she has done. Know the risks up front. Make an informed decision.

NOTE

1. Wood, M. Sandra. *Internet Guide to Cosmetic Surgery for Women*. Binghamton, NY: The Haworth Press, 2005.

Chapter 1

Cosmetic Plastic Surgery—The Facts

Have you been thinking about having a cosmetic surgery procedure done? Not sure whether you want to let friends and relatives know you are considering having that nose reshaped, the bags under your eyes removed, or those "love handles" removed? After all, isn't cosmetic surgery just for women—or is it?

Actually, you've seen some stories in the newspaper or on TV and know that, increasingly, more and more men are choosing to have cosmetic procedures. But, where do you start? Are you unsure about what is involved in the procedure—what you need to do to prepare for the surgery, what options are available, or how much "down time" is involved? Where do you find information, and what doctor should you choose? Maybe you don't want to ask anyone about cosmetic surgery because you don't know enough yet to ask intelligent questions?

Well, if any of these questions describe you, this book is just what you need to get started. A wealth of information is available via the Internet, and, it can be accessed anonymously. As cosmetic surgery becomes more "mainstream," the Internet is rapidly gaining popularity as the first resource to turn to for information. You can gather all sorts of background information about cosmetic surgery procedures, identify potential doctors to perform the procedures, and even chat online with others who have had cosmetic surgery, all from the comfort of your own home, via the Internet. In fact, there is too much information about cosmetic surgery on the Internet, and not all of it is accurate. This book is intended to guide you to quality sources of information about cosmetic surgery, but only you and a qualified physician can eventually make the decision as to whether or not you should undergo a cosmetic surgery procedure.

Internet Guide to Cosmetic Surgery for Men
© 2006 by The Haworth Press, Inc. All rights reserved.
doi:10.1300/5854_02

WHAT IS PLASTIC SURGERY?

Plastic surgery is the medical specialty involved with changing a person's appearance via surgery. Although people tend to think of plastic surgery in terms of its cosmetic use, in reality, according to the American Society of Plastic Surgeons, the majority of surgeries are reconstructive in nature. Cosmetic surgery is generally defined as surgery done for the purpose of improving appearance, i.e., it is plastic surgery for aesthetic purposes. Reconstructive surgery is done to correct or repair a defect, for example to correct a birth defect or repair an injury. The same procedure may be used either cosmetically or for reconstruction. Frequently, the purpose of the surgery determines whether it is covered by health insurance. Most cosmetic procedures are not covered by insurance, although it's always good to check with your health insurance company.

The primary focus of this book will be locating information about cosmetic procedures on the Internet. However, readers should keep in mind that a procedure may be used either for cosmetic or reconstructive purposes, so this book will also be valuable for those who need reconstructive surgery.

COSMETIC SURGERY IS A HOT TREND

Despite its cost, the days when cosmetic plastic surgery was limited to movie stars or the very rich and famous, are long gone. Gone, also, are the days when only women had cosmetic surgery; as you will see, the number of cosmetic procedures for men has increased dramatically.

Cosmetic surgery has boomed over the past decade or two, and several factors have contributed to this amazing increase in popularity. In recent years, people have become more open about having cosmetic surgery—it has become the "in" thing to do. Perhaps it's the aging baby-boomer set that doesn't want to admit it is aging; or, perhaps it's the increasing number of movie stars admitting—actually, being very public about the fact—that they have had cosmetic plastic surgery. The topic of cosmetic plastic surgery is much more out in the open than ever before. People that might not have considered cosmetic surgery several years ago are increasingly deciding to "go under the knife."

Cosmetic Surgery and Celebrities

The Internet is loaded with sites that discuss cosmetic surgery procedures of the stars. Several sites list the stars, what procedure was done, and before and after pictures.[1,2] Included are, to name only a few, Dick Clark, Tom Cruise, Michael Douglas, Paul Newman, Burt Reynolds, Arnold Schwarzenegger, and, of course, Michael Jackson. Yahoo! even has a "Celebrity Plastic Surgery" category among its directories.[3]

In fact, several sources go so far as to say that virtually everyone in Hollywood has had cosmetic surgery of some form or another. Although some are still reluctant to admit that they've had surgery, the fact is, in Tinsel-Town, looks are everything, and since age eventually takes its toll, cosmetic surgery, from laser peels through liposuction, ultimately wins out.[4]

In recent years, as more TV and movie stars have begun talking about their cosmetic procedures, "ordinary," everyday people are opening up about their experiences. Almost all of the daytime talk shows have explored the topic. It is constantly mentioned on syndicated TV shows such as *Entertainment Tonight (ET)* and *Extra,* and it's been discussed on many prime-time news shows and on ABC's *Good Morning America.*[5] In spring 2003, ABC TV introduced *Extreme Makeover* into its nighttime lineup of shows after the success of a pilot program in late 2002. This show takes ordinary people and offers them a free cosmetic surgery makeover. Application forms for people wanting to participate in this program can be found at <http://abc.go.com/primetime/extrememakeover/>. (*Note:* this is the form that will be used in this book for locations on the Internet. You will learn more about Internet addresses—URLs—in the next chapter.) Other networks are also offering shows about cosmetic surgery, including the FX network's *Nip/Tuck,* a show based on the life of a single, eligible plastic surgeon, and MTV's *I Want a Famous Face,* where patients undergo cosmetic surgery to look like a celebrity. Although these TV shows have popularized cosmetic surgery, many of the professional medical associations are concerned that the shows are unrealistic and do not disclose enough about the risks of surgery. TV shows such as *60 Minutes* and *20/20* have aired "exposés" about the risks of cosmetic surgery and the need to carefully select your surgeon.

Baby-Boomer Generation

As the generation of baby boomers has aged, health and physical fitness have become priorities. Men (and women) want to look and feel good about themselves. Cosmetic surgery is one way to keep a youthful appearance, whether it's used to erase those wrinkles and lines that appear with age, or to reshape one's body when exercise alone won't do the job.

Recent reports from the Centers for Disease Control indicate that obesity in America has become a major health concern. Interestingly, the increase in gastric bypass surgery (stomach stapling), a treatment for morbid obesity, has helped promote cosmetic surgical procedures. The major weight loss from stomach stapling can result in the need for cosmetic surgery to tighten up the body and remove excess skin.

More and more younger adults, even teens, are choosing to have plastic surgery as a means of correcting what they view as "defects" in their body. The prevailing attitude is, "if you don't like it, fix it." In the heavy-duty world of corporate America, "appearance is everything." The confidence gained as a result of cosmetic surgery might make the difference between being hired or not, or, between getting that promotion or not. In a culture that emphasizes youth, cosmetic surgery may give you that competitive edge in the workplace—or in luring a potential mate.[6]

WHAT ARE THE NUMBERS?

How many people have cosmetic surgery each year? What are the most frequent procedures, and how many men have certain procedures versus women? Does racial background play any part in cosmetic surgery? Is age a consideration? How much does it cost? These are all questions that come to mind when one is considering cosmetic surgery. After all, it is comforting to know that others have had the same cosmetic procedure that you are considering. Having some realistic expectation of both costs and results will help you to make your decision.

Answers to all of these questions, and more, can be found on the Internet. Perhaps the best source of statistics on cosmetic surgery is available on the Web site of the American Society of Plastic Surgeons (ASPS), <http://www.plasticsurgery.org>. Statistics are available on this site by year (currently, 1992 to 2004); by type of procedure; and by age, sex, and ethnicity. Also given are national average physicians' fees for cosmetic procedures (it's interesting to compare the most current year's average fees with earlier years). Some statistics reported are for procedures performed by "ASPS member plastic surgeons certified by The American Board of Plastic Surgery,"[7] while others include other ABMS-certified physicians.

The ASPS site includes many quick facts about cosmetic and reconstructive surgical and nonsurgical procedures. Press releases on the ASPS site for 2004 indicate that over 9.2 million cosmetic surgery procedures were performed in 2004, up 5 percent from 2002, and up 24 percent overall from 2000.

Looking only at cosmetic surgery procedures for men, according to the ASPS, there were 1.2 million cosmetic surgery procedures done for men in 2004; in fact, 13 percent of all cosmetic surgery patients were men. Also, according to the ASPS, the top five surgical procedures for men were nose reshaping (109,971), hair transplantation (43,054), eyelid surgery (32,667), liposuction (32,489), and breast reduction in men (13,963). The top five minimally invasive cosmetic procedures in men were Botox (329,187), microdermabrasion (214,717), laser hair removal (154,972), chemical peels (109,052), and collagen injections (31,306).

Another site that has excellent statistics for cosmetic surgery is the American Society for Aesthetic Plastic Surgery (ASAPS), <http://www.surgery.org>. According to the ASAPS, there were 11.9 million cosmetic procedures performed in the United States in 2004. Their statistics indicate that 10 percent of these procedures (1.2 million) were performed on men, with the top surgical procedures being liposuction (61,638), eyelid surgery (41,050), rhinoplasty (38,989), male breast reduction (19,636), and hair transplantation (19,503). The ASAPS reports the top five nonsurgical procedures are Botox injection (311,916), laser hair removal (196,847), chemical peels (133,124), microdermabrasion (99,221), and laser skin resurfacing (69,427).[8]

Many other sites on the Internet include statistics for cosmetic surgery, both in the United States and worldwide. However, the statistics available from these two associations will be listed for each procedure (where available) because of the structured reporting procedures for each group of physicians. Note that these statistics are updated each year by the ASPS and ASAPS, usually in February or March for the previous year.

If you are considering cosmetic surgery, you are definitely encouraged to log onto the ASPS site and the ASAPS site and check out the numbers—who's having what procedure done. It's reassuring to know that many, many other people have had the procedure(s) that you are considering.

HOW MUCH DOES IT COST?

One other really interesting piece of information provided by both the ASPS and ASAPS is the cost for cosmetic procedures. What is listed at each of these sites is the U.S. national average surgeon/physician fee. You should note that anesthesia, facilities (operating room, outpatient surgi-center), and other expenses are not included, and that variables such as geographic location are not included. In 2004, over $8.4 billion was spent on physicians' fees for cosmetic surgery according to the ASPS. For 2004, the ASAPS reports over $12.4 billion dollars spent.

WHY READ THIS BOOK?

Every person—man or woman—wants to feel good about himself or herself. A positive self concept is linked to how you look and feel. How you look can be enhanced by cosmetic surgery. The decision to have cosmetic plastic surgery is a big step. It involves a physical change that will alter not only how you will look at yourself, but also how others will look at you. There are risks with surgery. Surgical costs are normally not covered by health insurance—all factors to consider.

As you begin to evaluate whether or not you might want to undergo cosmetic surgery, you should gather as much information as possible so that you can make an informed decision. Although many people have had cosmetic surgery, you might not know anyone who can tell you of their experience. Even if you know someone who has had a cosmetic procedure, you might not feel comfortable asking him or her about it. Locally, you will find that many plastic surgeons hold clinics to explain procedures. These informational meetings are usually a way of advertising and promoting procedures at their clinics. Even before attending such a meeting, knowing what is involved in a cosmetic procedure will help you to evaluate and ask good questions.

This is where the Internet comes in to play. Besides the information that your doctor will give to you, the Internet is perhaps your best source for information about cosmetic procedures. However, the Internet can be overwhelming because of the quantity of information—Web sites are plentiful and chat groups abound. There is so much available that it can be confusing, not all of it is accurate, and some sites can be misleading. This book will help you to identify Internet resources you can trust. The following chapters will cover basic Internet searching, finding a doctor, and how to locate information about specific cosmetic surgical and non-surgical (minimally invasive) procedures. You'll learn about evaluating information from a Web site, selecting a "credentialed" physician, and locating information about specific procedures.

Ultimately, the choice of whether or not to have cosmetic surgery is yours, and yours alone. Input of family and friends and your doctor will all influence your decision, but the better informed you are about the surgical procedure, along with risks and complications, the better your decision. Resources in this book are intended to lead you to quality information to help you in your decision-making process. Keep in mind, though, that the information found in this book and on the Internet is not a substitute for the advice of your cosmetic surgeon, who is best qualified to evaluate you (your medical/physical condition) and determine whether you are a candidate for the cosmetic procedure you wish to have.

NOTES

1. Plastic People Page. Available: <http://www.geocities.com/hollywood/7990/plastic. html>. Accessed: October 7, 2005.

2. "Hollywood and Cosmetic Surgery. Available: <http://www.streamingsurgeries. com/hollywood/cosmetic_surgery_hollywood.html>. Accessed: October 7, 2005.

3. Yahoo! "Celebrity Plastic Surgery." Available: <http://www.yahoo.com.>Directory >Culture >People >Celebrities >Plastic Surgery>. Accessed: October 7, 2005.

4. "Looking Like a Celebrity. Plastic Surgery at the Front Lines of Glamour." ABC News.com. Available: <http://printerfriendly.abcnews.com/printerfriendly/Print?fetch FromGLUE=trueandGLUESer...>. Accessed: May 28, 2003.

5. Pozniak, Alexa. "Face Off Over Face-Lifts. Experts Say 'Not So Fast' to Face-Lifts for 30-Somethings." ABCNews.com Available: <http://printerfriendly.abcnews.com/ printerfriendly/Print?fetchFromGLUE=trueandGLUESer...>. Accessed: May 28, 2003 [no longer available].

6. CNN.com. "Look Who's Going Under the Knife: Men and Plastic Surgery." (October 25, 1999). Available: <http://www.cnn.com/HEALTH/men/9910/25/plastic.surgery. men.wmd/>. Accessed: October 14, 2005.

7. American Society of Plastic Surgeons. Available: <http://www.plasticsurgery.org>.

8. American Society for Aesthetic Plastic Surgery. Available: <http://www.surgery. org>.

Chapter 2

The Internet—A Brief Look at Where to Begin

Finding information about cosmetic surgery on the Internet is easy. Finding quality information on the Internet is a bit trickier. In fact, finding too much information on the Internet is, perhaps, the biggest problem. Literally millions of "hits" come up when doing a general search on "cosmetic surgery" or "plastic surgery" using the search feature of two of the major search engines, Internet Explorer and Netscape. Hundreds of thousands of sites can be located on individual procedures such as liposuction and Botox. The amount of information available is absolutely mind-boggling and extremely confusing. In fact, it is so confusing that you may be tempted to simply give up before you really start. The idea of having to wade through thousands of sites can be a real turnoff to continuing your search.

This is where knowing where to start searching and how to locate the best Web sites becomes valuable both in terms of time and quality of information. It's really important to be selective in what you look at on the Net. Using the simple tips listed in this chapter, along with going to the sites targeted later in this book, will give you the necessary know-how to find accurate information about cosmetic procedures that you're interested in and will also help you to find a qualified physician located near you.

THE INTERNET

This book assumes a basic knowledge of the Internet—that you know it is a large, worldwide computer network (actually, it's a network of networks) that allows users to access information from around the world. Some basic information about Web addresses (hyperlinked sites on the

Internet Guide to Cosmetic Surgery for Men
© 2006 by The Haworth Press, Inc. All rights reserved.
doi:10.1300/5854_03

Internet) will be given in this book. If you are a new Internet user ("newbie") and need more extensive information about the Net, you are advised to consult a basic Internet search guide such as *The Internet for Dummies*.[1] The second assumption is that you, the reader, have access to the Internet either at home or work, through a public library, from an Internet café, or through some other location.

INTERNET ADDRESSES

The Internet and the World Wide Web (WWW, or simply "the Web") are not the same thing, although many people use these terms interchangeably. The Web uses a system of links between documents, or pages of information, that have been placed on a computer using hypertext markup language (html). The set of standards for linking to these documents is called hypertext transfer protocol (http), which is the prefix that you will see listed at the beginning of most Internet addresses. The locations for these documents, called "Web sites," are given addresses, known as URLs—for uniform resource locators. Throughout this book, you will see URLs listed in a standard format, consisting of the document format or protocol (http), followed by the host computer, directory, and file name, surrounded by angle brackets to set off the address. It will appear like this:

<protocol://host.domain.suffix/directory/file.extension>

For example, in the address

<http://www.nlm.nih.gov/medlineplus/plasticandcosmeticsurgery.html>,

the protocol is http, which tells you that it is a Web page; this is followed by ://www, which tells you this is a Web address; the domain is the National Library of Medicine at the National Institutes of Health, which is a government agency (.gov); the directory is MedlinePlus; the file name is plastic and cosmeticsurgery; and the file extension is html.

MY SITE IS GONE!

As you begin searching the Internet, you need to remember that the Web is "fluid"—sites are constantly being updated, changed, added, and deleted, all of which leads to outdated sites and dead links. Dead links are the result of a change to a file name or site address. You may have been given the address of a good Web site to start your search, and after you type in the URL, you get a message that the site or page can't be found. Frequently, if it's just the page that has been removed, you will be redirected to the main, or home page. However, when you encounter a dead or broken link and you are not redirected, you should delete information at the end of the address—e.g., the /directory, /filename.htm, or /filename.html part of the address—and use only the host.domain.suffix part of the address (e.g., <http://www.nlm.nih.gov>). From there, you can search the site for the specific Web page or document or topic that you are looking for. If you still cannot access the site, the whole site may have changed addresses, in which case you would need to do a Net search as described in "Searching via Your Internet Browser" in this chapter.

Another way to locate information that has "disappeared" from the Internet is to go to the Wayback Machine <http://www.archive.org/web/web.php>. This site has a simple search interface that locates archived Web pages back to 1996.

EVALUATING WEB SITES: THE "GOOD" VERSUS THE "BAD"

Whether you are an experienced computer user, or someone just getting started with the Internet, some cautions are in order. A general subject search on cosmetic surgery using any Internet browser will bring up hundreds of thousands of "hits"—sites that presumably include some information on cosmetic surgery. Unfortunately, the sites that appear on the list first may not be the "best" sites. In fact, the first sites that appear may have paid to have their site listed first or in a prominent location. Sites that look relevant and appear attractive may actually contain biased, incorrect, or even dangerous information. Anyone can create a Web site that appears authoritative—from a professional organization to a doctor's office practice to your teenage son. As you scroll down the screen looking at the sites you've located, you may find that many sites are repeated, some look irrelevant, and a few may even be totally inappropriate sites—some terminology in cosmetic surgery may actually lead you to pornographic sites.

So, how do you choose which sites to look at? Once you click the hyperlink to go to the site, how do you determine whether the site you've just connected to has "good" information? At minimum, quality, authoritative Web sites should be evaluated for the following:

- *Who created the site?* The person or group responsible for the content should be identified, along with a way to contact them by e-mail, fax, mail, or telephone. Credentials of the creator should be listed (e.g., education, experience, institutional affiliation) so that you can determine credibility.
- *Currency/last update.* How well maintained is this site? The last update of the site should be listed; sites not frequently updated should be skipped. Are links to other sites still working?
- *Seal of approval.* Several national and international organizations have been created to accredit Web sites. One such organization is the Health on the Net Foundation (HON) at <http://www.hon.ch>. HON is an international Swiss organization that guides Internet searchers to reliable and useful medical and health information. Web sites given HON approval are classified as educational, individual, or commercial. The Utilization Review Accreditation Commission (URAC), <http://websiteaccreditation.urac.org>, is an American organization that accredits quality health Web sites.
- *Bias.* Sites that give only one viewpoint (e.g., discuss a cosmetic procedure without listing risks) should be avoided. Does the site sell products or advertise a physician's clinic? Is it sponsored by a drug company?
- *Intended audience.* Web sites may be created for medical professionals (physicians, nurses) or for consumers (e.g., patients, prospective patients, general public).
- *Look at the domain name.* The Web site address itself can be helpful in evaluating a site. The ending of the address indicates the location, e.g., ".gov" is a U.S. government site, ".org" is an organization, and ".edu" is an educational institution (however, a tilde or "~" in the ".edu" address indicates personal Web space within the educational institution and could be a student's Web site). The country of origin can be determined by the site's URL, for example, .au indicates an Australian site, .ca is a Canadian site, and .uk is a United Kingdom site.

- *Presentation/content.* Does the Web site look like it was put together in haste—i.e., are there a lot of typographical errors? Is it easy to navigate? Are pages linked logically? Overall, how well is it presented graphically?

Not all of these points must be present in a Web site for it to be considered a good or valuable site, but if in doubt, use these guidelines to evaluate how trustworthy it is.

Sites selected for inclusion in this book have been evaluated by the author based on the previous criteria. Not all of the sites selected meet all of the criteria. An attempt was made to select sites with quality content that would be representative of the types of sites found on the Internet, including organizations, government, and commercial sites.

BASIC INTERNET SEARCHING

Each individual seems to have a favorite way to search the Internet. Some people just use the "Search" feature on their browser (e.g., Internet Explorer, Netscape), and input a search term (e.g., liposuction). Others have a favorite search engine, such as Google, Mamma, or Yahoo!. Still others have favorite megasites that they've bookmarked in special subject areas (e.g., MedlinePlus might be bookmarked for medicine and health care information). Although each of these methods might provide some useful information, a combination is the best approach. Methods described in this chapter include:

- Searching via your Internet browser
- Searching via a search engine/directory
- Searching via megasites

Of these methods, searching megasites is preferable. However, since most people are more likely to be familiar with search engines or using their Internet browser, those will be briefly described first, followed by several recommended megasites to be used as starting points. Ultimately, though, you will be encouraged to use the recommended sites in later chapters of this book.

SEARCHING VIA YOUR INTERNET BROWSER

Internet browsers such as Netscape and Internet Explorer each have a "Search" feature that allows you to input a search term and get a list of "hits" on your topic. Subscribers to commercial services such as America Online (AOL) will also find a search feature on their home page. Although this appears to be the easiest method for finding information, it is the least recommended, and potentially, the most hazardous. For example, this author recently searched Netscape (which features Google) using "cosmetic surgery"—and found too many "hits" to look through. "Sponsored Links" appeared first (links that pay to be at the top), followed by "Matching Results"—in no particular order, although there were a high number of .com sites (commercial sites). Searching for "plastic surgery," "liposuction," and "Botox" brought up similarly lengthy lists. Clearly, the amount of information is overwhelming. How would you make a good choice on what links to follow, what sites to access? This is definitely *not* recommended as the best way to begin, but I recognize that many people will start here almost by default. However, several alternatives are available.

SEARCHING VIA A SEARCH ENGINE/DIRECTORY

Many search engines are available on the Internet. A search engine can either be man-made or a robot—a computer doing the search based on pre-programming. These search engines can be used in two ways. The first method is similar to a Web browser, where you simply enter a word or phrase. A recent search of "cosmetic surgery" in Google, a popular search engine, resulted in 11,300,000 "hits"—so many sites that it was impossible to make a good selection of what site to visit. The number of sites found represents exponential growth in the sites available on cosmetic surgery, as the "hits" were nearly three times the number found just one year earlier, and that number was almost three times larger than the year before.

Some of the more popular search engines are listed in Table 2.1. However, be forewarned that use of these engines will result in extensive lists of "hits" on cosmetic surgery sites, often in no particular order other than sponsored sites being listed first. Although some good sites might be found this way, it soon becomes both boring and frustrating to try to filter out good sites to view. There are simply so many commercial and special interest sites to sort through that it's difficult to identify quality information.

TABLE 2.1. Selected Search Engines

Search Engine	URL
AlltheWeb	<http://www.alltheweb.com>
Alta Vista	<http://www.altavista.com>
Ask Jeeves	<http://www.ask.com>
Dogpile	<http://www.dogpile.com>
Google	<http://www.google.com>
HotBot	<http://www.hotbot.com>
Ixquick Metasearch	<http://www.ixquick.com>
LookSmart	<http://www.looksmart.com>
Mamma	<http://www.mamma.com>
MetaCrawler	<http://www.metacrawler.com>
Teoma	<http://www.teoma.com>
Vivisimo	<http://www.vivisimo.com>
Yahoo!	<http://www.yahoo.com>

Search engines/directories vary in size and how they are organized, updated, and searched. No attempt will be made to give detailed instruction on how to search each engine. Rather, only simple searches—one word or a brief phrase—are recommended. Detailed information about complex search strategies can be found at Search Engine Showdown <http://www.searchengineshowdown.com/? and Search Engine Watch <http://searchenginewatch.com/>. The intent here is to keep search topics as simple as possible, e.g., "cosmetic surgery," "liposuction," etc.

Some of the search engines have directories that have been created to gather together information on general subject areas. For example, directory searching is available on Google and Yahoo! Vivisimo has something called "Clusters" that serve a similar function as a directory. Several of my favorite search engines are briefly described, and Table 2.1 has a longer list of selected search engines. Keep in mind, though, that better ways of finding information on cosmetic surgery and more specific procedures are given later in this book.

Dogpile
<http://www.dogpile.com>

Dogpile bills itself as "all the best search engines piled into one." As a metasearch engine, it searches many resources at one time, including Google, Ask Jeeves, and Yahoo! This advantage can also be a disadvantage, as almost any search brings back a large number of "hits." Sponsored links are clearly marked and appear on the line with the hot link; sponsored sites are listed before all others.

Google
<http://www.google.com>

Google is a favorite search engine of librarians and physicians. In fact, most people are familiar with the phrase, "to Google someone." Googling has become an American slang word. In addition to its general search capability, Google also has a directory <http://directory.google.com/> that you can browse and search. Google is one of the largest search engines, and links to Web sites, discussion/news groups, images, and more. Cosmetic surgery is buried deep within the directory. To reach it, select "Google Directory," then "Health," then "Medicine," then "Surgery," and finally "Cosmetic and Plastic." However, once you've reached this level, access points include directories (listings of physicians), organizations, patient education (procedures), and surgeons and clinics. The surgeons and clinics section is organized by country, and within the United States, by state; links here go to physicians' individual Web sites.

Vivisimo
<http://www.vivisimo.com>

Vivisimo is a meta-search engine, meaning it searches several search engines at once. A search on "cosmetic surgery" brought up over 8.5 million hits. A great feature of Visisimo is its clustering. Despite the large number of hits, it clusters like topics together, offering a link to a cluster of sites on laser surgery or facial plastic surgery, for example.

Yahoo!
<http://www.yahoo.com>

As with the other search engines, you can enter your search term directly into a "search box" and click "go." To access the Yahoo! Directory, scroll to the Web Site Directory, and from there choose "Health," then "Procedures and Therapies," then "Surgeries," and then "Cosmetic and Plastic." Links are available for selected cosmetic procedures. Just for fun, you can also locate information on celebrities having plastic surgery from the "Web Site Directory" on Yahoo!'s home page by selecting "Culture," then "People," then "Celebrities," and finally "Plastic Surgery."

SEARCHING VIA A MEGASITE

The recommended way to begin searching on the Internet for information about cosmetic surgery procedures is to begin with a megasite. A megasite is defined here as a site that contains large amounts of information or links to information on other Web sites. These sites do not create the information, but provide organized access to information on other Web sites. The sites listed as follows were selected from a group of excellent resources. It's just not possible to include an exhaustive list. The resources and links included in these sites will get you started in the right direction—gathering quality information to help you make a decision about whether or not to have a cosmetic surgical procedure.

Ask NOAH About: Plastic and Cosmetic Surgery
<http://www.noah-health.org>

NOAH (New York Online Access to Health) is a megasite created by a cooperative of libraries in New York City. Originally intended as a guide to health care information for residents of New York City, this resource has grown into a major site recognized worldwide as providing quality health information. From the main NOAH page, select "Health Topics" and then "Plastic Surgery," or go directly to <http://www.noah-health.org/en/procedures/surgery/cosmetic/>. On this page (see Figure 2.1) are links to information about specific procedures; definitions; complications, including insurance and safety issues; care and treatment; and information resources. Most links go to consumer sites provided by professional orga-

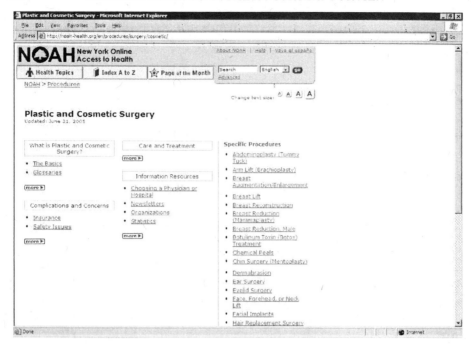

FIGURE 2.1. NOAH Page on Plastic and Reconstructive Surgery
<http://noah-health.org/en/procedures/surgery/cosmetic/>
Reprinted with permission of New York Online Access to Health.

nizations and university health centers; all resources have been evaluated by librarians before being linked into the NOAH page. This is a great place to start your search for quality information, and it also contains links to resources for choosing a physician or a hospital. A Spanish version of NOAH is available.

MedlinePlus
<http://medlineplus.gov>

MedlinePlus is made available by the National Library of Medicine (NLM), the world's largest medical library. It is "designed to help you find appropriate, authoritative health information" at both the consumer and professional level. The site contains health news, drug information, an illustrated medical encyclopedia, a dictionary, links to medical databases such as MEDLINE, and links to other Web sites containing health information on over 600 diseases. NLM clearly posts its selection guidelines for these materials, including quality of content, noncommercial sources, and availability/maintenance of the Web pages. This site is considered to be the premier Web site for consumer health materials, and thus is an excellent starting place for locating information on cosmetic and plastic surgery.

Once in MedlinePlus, select "Health Topics" and then the letter "P." On the "P" page, select "Plastic & Cosmetic Surgery." This page brings together the majority of links in MedlinePlus about cosmetic surgery (see Figure 2.2). From the latest news and general information through links to specific procedures, treatment, and statistics, this page is a great place to start gathering information about the cosmetic procedures that interest you. A majority of the links on this page go to pages produced for consumers by professional organizations, including the American Society of Plastic Surgeons and the American Academy of Facial Plastic and Reconstructive

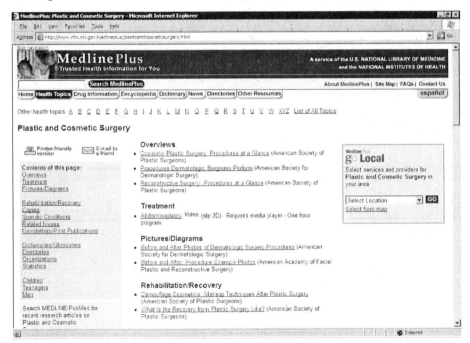

FIGURE 2.2. MedlinePlus Page on Plastic and Cosmetic Surgery
<http://www.nlm.nih.gov/medlineplus/plasticandcosmeticsurgery.html>

Surgery (more on these later in this book). From this page, you can also link to other relevant MedlinePlus pages on topics such as Botox, breast implants, scars, and varicose veins. A Spanish version of MedlinePlus is available, also.

MOVING ON TO SPECIFIC SITES

As you begin to become familiar with the primary sites that are linked to these megasites, you will then begin to recognize them as authoritative and go directly to those sites. For example, you will find that sites such as the American Society of Plastic Surgeons and the American Society for Aesthetic Plastic Surgery will be prominently featured within these megasites, along with other professional organizations, government sites, and some commercial sites. You will then be ready to begin looking for information on specific procedures at the specific sites listed in later chapters of this book.

NOTE

1. Levine, John, Young, Margaret Levine, and Baroudi, Carol. *The Internet for Dummies,* Tenth Edition. Hoboken, NJ: Wiley Publishing, 2005 (or later edition).

Chapter 3

Checking Out Credentials

As you evaluate whether to have cosmetic surgery, you will need to learn about procedures that are available and to make a decision on who will perform your cosmetic surgery. If you are anxious to begin learning about the procedures, then skip ahead to later chapters in this book, where you will find Internet sites about many popular cosmetic surgery procedures. However, many of the recommended sites are, in fact, produced for prospective patients (consumers such as yourself) by the professional membership associations of cosmetic surgeons, so it's important that you understand the role these organizations play in certifying that your prospective surgeon has the proper training and experience to perform cosmetic procedures. This chapter will help you to select a cosmetic surgeon by leading you to information about both the selection process and physician credentials. So, while you may actually decide first on what cosmetic procedure you want, understanding the qualifications and medical/surgical specialties and subspecialties that are involved with cosmetic surgery may actually influence the procedure that you ultimately select. A "good fit" between you and your surgeon will lead to a positive experience.

HOW TO FIND A GOOD COSMETIC SURGEON

You may already be at the point where you have a surgeon in mind. For example, you might have looked in your local phone book, checked the yellow pages, and made a selection based on what's listed in the doctor's ad. In fact, you may have already checked out several prospective surgeons

Internet Guide to Cosmetic Surgery for Men
© 2006 by The Haworth Press, Inc. All rights reserved.
doi:10.1300/5854_04

on the Internet because many doctors' offices list their Web address (URL) in the phone book or newspaper ads, and maybe you've gone online to their Web site. It has become fairly routine now for doctors to place Web site information in the local yellow pages just so potential patients (like you) can check information online in the privacy of their own homes.

Maybe you know someone who has had plastic surgery and you asked whether or not they would recommend the physician who performed the surgery. Person-to-person referral is still one of the best ways to locate potential surgeons. You can get firsthand information about how your friend felt about his or her experience from comments about the doctor to whether any problems or difficulties occurred following the surgery. You also have an opportunity to see how the surgery actually turned out. After all, cosmetic surgery is a very personal decision, and you will need to feel comfortable with both the surgeon and the results of the surgery.

The recent development of the Internet has greatly expanded your capability to locate and select a cosmetic surgeon, both locally and at a distance. Although most people will select a local surgeon, you can now use the Internet to find an expert worldwide should you decide that you want to travel to another location for your surgery.

Some basic guidelines to consider in selecting a cosmetic surgeon:

- Check your surgeon's credentials. Board certification, medical licensure, and membership in professional organizations are all relevant to how well your surgeon is qualified.
- What surgery center/hospital does your surgeon use? Is it accredited?
- Check your surgeon's malpractice history.
- How many years has your surgeon been practicing? How many procedures has he or she done of the type you are considering?
- Ask to see examples (photos) of the work that he or she has done.
- Do you feel comfortable with this surgeon? How well does he or she listen to what you say you want done? Does he or she answer all of your questions?

The Internet has many sites that actually provide checklists and questions for you to ask your prospective surgeon. A few are briefly listed as follows, with more detailed descriptions of these and other Web sites in later chapters of this book.

**American Academy of Cosmetic Surgery—How to Choose
a Cosmetic Surgeon**
<http://www.cosmeticsurgery.org/Patients/choosingasurgeon.asp>

**American Society of Plastic Surgeons—How to Choose a Plastic
Surgeon**
<http://www.plasticsurgery.org/find_a_plastic_surgeon/How-to-
Choose-a-Plastic-Surgeon.cfm>

**Facial Plastic Surgery Network—How to Find & Choose a Great
Surgeon**
<http://www.facialplasticsurgery.net/findingasurgeon.htm>

Yes They're Fake!—Surgeon Information
<http://www.yestheyrefake.net/plastic_surgeon?information.htm>

CREDENTIALS/BOARD CERTIFICATION

Much of the decision process depends on personal opinion and a certain comfort level. Perhaps more important, though, is the need to evaluate the credentials of the doctor who will perform your cosmetic procedure. Cosmetic surgery requires special training and certification by appropriate "boards" before a physician is considered to be fully qualified. One of the main credentials that you will see listed for a physician is that the doctor is "board certified." Having a medical degree (MD or DO) is not enough. What is the physician's specialty? Would you want a radiologist to perform liposuction? Or, would you feel comfortable with your family physician performing breast enlargement? The radiologist and family physician will be board certified in their own specialty, but that does not qualify them to perform cosmetic plastic surgery. Thus, a physician indicating that he or she is "board certified" is insufficient information for you to make a decision. What board has certified them?

In recent years, as cosmetic plastic surgery has become more popular, physicians who are board certified in other specialties have taken quick courses on cosmetic surgery and begun to perform cosmetic procedures. They don't need to deal with insurance companies for reimbursement (after all, you are paying for the procedures and they can charge what they want), and this has become a way to increase/augment their income. Although these physicians may do a fine job, you should be fully aware of a physician's qualifications and track record before undergoing any surgical procedure.

ABMS Board Certification

Board certification implies a basic knowledge and skill level, frequently determined by a number of years of postgraduate medical training and experience (residency), passing an examination, and maintaining skills through continuing education. When searching for a qualified physician, evaluating credentials such as board certification is essential. However, there is not just one board that certifies physicians who perform cosmetic procedures, and this can be very confusing as you evaluate credentials.

The American Board of Medical Specialists (ABMS) is an organization made up of twenty-four approved medical specialty boards that grant certification to physicians (MDs and DOs) who have completed an approved training program (residency) and passed an examination. Similar boards approve specialty training in other countries around the world. Although you will find board-certified physicians from many specialties offering cosmetic procedures, you should look for a physician certified by one of the following specialty boards to perform your cosmetic plastic surgery: American Board of Plastic Surgery, American Board of Dermatology, American Board of Ophthalmology, American Board of Otolaryngology, and American Board of Surgery. Physicians from other medical specialties may also perform certain types of cosmetic surgery.

You can check out board certification for any of the ABMS specialties by going to its Web site at <http://www.abms.org>. Select the link, "Who's Certified." You will need to register (it's free), and once registered, you can check out specific individuals' names for board certification. More complete information about using the ABMS directory can be found at <http://www.abms.org>, along with links to each specialty board.

Other boards also exist for subspecialties (e.g., cosmetic surgery and facial cosmetic surgery); they represent further specialization and often are listed as qualifications by cosmetic surgeons in addition to the ABMS board certification. In the following descriptions, the American Board of Plastic Surgery is listed first, with the other specialties then listed alphabetically. Information about other selected specialty/subspecialty boards follows.

American Board of Plastic Surgery
<http://www.abplsurg.org/>

The mission of the ABPS is to "promote safe, ethical, efficacious plastic surgery to the public by maintaining high standards for the examination and certification of plastic surgeons as specialists and subspecialists." Information about the board-certification process and examination information is available. This site is primarily for physicians specializing in plastic surgery, but is of interest to health care consumers because standards are listed. The ABPS is a member organization of the American Board of Medical Specialists and is the primary certifying body in the United States for plastic surgeons. Within this site, you can find the criteria for certification, which include an MD or DO degree, completion of an accredited residency program, and passing an examination. More complete information is available on the ABPS Web site. To check out board certification, you are referred to the ABMS Web site <http://www.abms.org>. Select "Who's Certified" and follow the registration directions (it's free). In addition to being board certified in plastic surgery, you would also want your surgeon to be a member of a professional association such as the American Society of Plastic Surgeons (ASPS) or the American Society for Aesthetic Plastic Surgery.

American Board of Dermatology
<http://www.abderm.org>

The American Board of Dermatology is accredited by the ABMS to certify physicians as specialists in dermatology. Dermatologists must complete postgraduate training and pass an examination to become board certified. Dermatologists evaluate and treat patients with "disorders of the skin, hair, nails and adjacent mucous membranes." According to this site, "Dermatologists also manage cosmetic disorders of the skin, including hair loss, scars, and the skin changes associated with aging." Thus, many dermatologists will perform cosmetic procedures involving the skin and face.

If you select "Verifying Certification" you are taken to a page that gives directions for mailing $35.00 to the ABD for written verification. Instead, for free verification, follow the link at the bottom to the ABMS Web listings, or call the number listed for verbal verification. If you are looking for a physician to perform a cosmetic skin procedure, in addition to being certified in dermatology, you will want to look for credentials like membership in an organization such as the American Society for Dermatologic Surgery and the American Academy of Dermatology.

American Board of Ophthalmology
<http://www.abop.org>

The American Board of Ophthalmology certifies ophthalmologists in the United States. The ABO page refers you to the ABMS page <http://www.abms.org> for online verification of certified ophthalmologists (free, but you must register), and provides directions for obtaining written verification (for a fee). In addition to being certified by the ABO, you would also want your physician to be a member of the American Society of Ophthalmic Plastic & Reconstructive Surgery, which requires further specialization.

American Board of Otolaryngology
<http://www.aboto.org>

The American Board of Otolaryngology (ABOto) is the organization recognized by the ABMS to certify otolaryngologists, the specialty that deals with head and neck surgery. Cosmetic and reconstructive plastic surgery of the head and neck may be performed by an otolaryngologist. From this site, you can click on diplomat verification and get free online verification. You would also want your surgeon to be a member of an organization such as the American Academy of Facial Plastic and Reconstructive Surgery, or certified by the American Board of Facial Plastic and Reconstructive Surgery, which requires further specialization.

American Board of Surgery
<http://www.absurgery.org>

"The ABS is an independent, non-profit organization with worldwide recognition. It is one of the twenty-four certifying boards that are members of the American Board of Medical Specialties." To check on board certification for your physician, you are directed to link to the ABMS Web site, or to make your inquiry via mail or phone to the ABS. Since this board certifies general surgeons, you would want your surgeon to have further specialization and training in cosmetic surgery, for example with one of the subspecialty boards mentioned in the next section, depending on the specific type of procedures that he or she performs.

Dental Board

American Board of Oral and Maxillofacial Surgery
<http://www.aboms.org>

"The American Board of Oral and Maxillofacial Surgery (ABOMS) is the certifying board for the specialty of oral and maxillofacial surgery in the United States and is recognized and approved by the Council on Dental Education of the American Dental Association." This organization certifies dentists who specialize in oral surgery, which includes cosmetic dentistry and cosmetic surgery of the maxillofacial area. Certification can be verified (select "Verifications" from the main page and then you must have the dentist's social security number), but there is a fee of $25.00 per verification.

Subspecialty Boards

American Board of Cosmetic Surgery
<http://www.americanboardcosmeticsurgery.org>

Founded in 1979 as the American Board of Aesthetic Plastic Surgery, the American Board of Cosmetic Surgery states that its mission is "to serve the public by promoting the safe and ethical practice of the specialty of cosmetic surgery. Diplomats of the ABCS shall demonstrate the highest standards of training, knowledge, and expertise, as determined by a process of peer review and standardized examination and certification." Candidates for certification by the ABCS must meet rigorous criteria that include proof of prior board certification by one of five specialties recognized by the ABMS, the Bureau of Osteopathic Specialists of the American Osteopathic Association, or the Royal College of Physicians and Surgeons of Canada, or certification by the American Board of Oral and Maxillofacial Surgery; 150 CME credits in cosmetic surgery in the three years prior to application; successful completion of a written examination covering cosmetic surgical procedures; and more. There are currently more than 400 ABCS members in the United States and worldwide, with a growing membership.

Although this Web site is aimed at the practicing cosmetic surgeon, patients can use the Directory on the left-hand side of the main page to locate ABCS diplomats by name in the alphabetic "ABCS Diplomates Index," or geographically by the "Geographic search." The list gives basic information (name, degrees, location), but if the surgeon has a Web site, a hot link can be used to access the doctor's site.

American Board of Facial Plastic and Reconstructive Surgery
<http://www.abfprs.org/>

Some plastic surgeons limit their practice primarily to cosmetic, plastic, or reconstructive surgery of the face. The American Board of Facial Plastic and Reconstructive Surgery (ABFPRS), established in 1986, is "dedicated to improving the quality of facial plastic surgery available to the public by measuring the qualifications of candidate surgeons against certain rigorous standards." To achieve certification by the ABFPRS, the surgeon must have completed an accredited residency program with training in facial plastic surgery, and be certified by the American Board of Plastic Surgery and/or the American Board of Otolaryngology, or in Canada, the Royal College of Physicians and Surgeons of Canada in otolaryngology or plastic surgery. In addition, he or she must pass a special examination, and also present "100 surgical cases in facial plastic and reconstructive surgery for each of the previous two years."

Part of this Web site is aimed at physicians interested in becoming certified by the ABFPRS. However, if you select "Who's Certified" at the top of the page, you can access the list of certified facial plastic surgeons. Simply click to "accept" the disclaimer at the bottom of the page (absolves the board of liability), and you are directed to a page where you can select your state, or state and physician name. You can view all ABFPRS certified physicians in your state, or look for a specific physician. Name, city, and phone number are given for all physicians, along with a link to the physician's Web site, if one is available.

Professional Membership Organizations

There are many professional membership organizations that cosmetic plastic surgeons elect or qualify to join. Membership in such an organization carries with it both prestige and an implied level of competence. Many membership organizations, such as the American Society of Plastic Surgeons, require that members be board certified and have taken additional continuing education courses to be a member. You will want your surgeon to be both board certified and a member of a professional organization related to cosmetic surgery.

Web sites of these membership organizations are featured throughout this book because they provide information to prospective patients about cosmetic surgery procedures and offer free doctor-locator services. These organizations' Web sites also give advice on how to evaluate and select a cosmetic surgeon, so these sites are featured as physician selection sites (see next section). A more comprehensive description of the Web sites of these organizations will appear in Chapter 4, "Basic/Core Sites on Cosmetic Surgery."

LOCATING/SELECTING A COSMETIC SURGEON ONLINE

The Web abounds with sites that claim to be able to locate cosmetic surgeons throughout the United States and worldwide. As you look through the Internet, and in fact with some commercial sites listed in this book, many sites claim to have a "physician locator." Use of commercial sites to locate your cosmetic surgeon is *not* recommended. In fact, if you decide to explore these sites, you will often find only one or two physicians listed per state, limiting the usefulness of these sites. Rather, you should limit your search for a qualified cosmetic surgeon to listings in professional membership organizations. In general, Web sites of professional organizations have the best, most comprehensive, and up-to-date physician-locator lists—as you would expect, since cosmetic surgeons want to be able to list membership in these organizations as one of their credentials. Table 3.1 shows a selected list of U.S. cosmetic surgery associations that offer physician-locator information. Although they are U.S. based, some of them have Canadian and/or worldwide membership. The most comprehensive listing is the Plastic Surgeon Referral Service of the American Society of Plastic Surgeons.

Rather than duplicate listings, each of these sites will be described in detail in Chapter 4. A selected list of organizations from other countries is given in Chapter 11 for non-U.S. readers, or for U.S. readers who are contemplating surgery outside the United States.

TABLE 3.1. Professional Organization Web Sites with Physician Locators

Organization/URL	From Home Page Select:
American Academy of Cosmetic Surgery <http://www.cosmeticsurgery.org>	Patient Information > Surgeon Finder
American Academy of Dermatology <http://www.aad.org>	Find a Dermatologist
American Academy of Facial Plastic and Reconstructive Surgery <http://www.aafprs.org>	Patients > Physician Finder
American Society for Aesthetic Plastic Surgery <http://www.surgery.org>	Find a Surgeon
American Society for Dermatologic Surgery <http://www.asds-net.org>	Find a Dermatologic Surgeon
American Society of Ophthalmic Plastic and Reconstructive Surgeons <http://www.asoprs.org>	Membership > Membership Directory
American Society of Plastic Surgeons <http://www.plasticsurgery.org>	Find a Plastic Surgeon

NEXT: BASIC COSMETIC SURGERY SITES ON THE INTERNET

So, you've made a preliminary decision about that surgeon you might wish to perform your cosmetic surgery procedure. But, you want to know more about the procedure that you *think* you want and what alternatives might be available. When you go for a preliminary meeting with your surgeon, you want to know enough to ask the right questions and to understand his or her answers. In short, you want to be knowledgeable and informed. Chapter 4 will get you started with an overview of basic sites about cosmetic surgery.

Chapter 4

Basic/Core Sites on Cosmetic Surgery

This chapter focuses on basic, core Web sites that provide information on cosmetic surgery procedures. Several male-only sites are featured, but they are rare. Despite the growing popularity of cosmetic surgery among men, most of the sites seem to be aimed at women. Remember, however, that many procedures are similar in men and women.

Out of the hundreds of thousands of sites available, relatively few could be selected for this book. Selection was primarily based on criteria listed in Chapter 1 for evaluating information on the Internet, including reputation of the source, currency, nonbiased information, and presentation. Many of the selected sites are produced by U.S. professional associations (.org); these sites often feature membership information that will help you to locate a cosmetic surgeon in your area. It was impossible to ignore the highly commercial nature of cosmetic surgery, which is reflected in the large number of commercial sites on the Internet. Some of these commercial sites are quite well done and provide extensive, unique, and relevant information. Therefore, selected, representative commercial sites are included where it was felt that it would help you make an informed decision about your cosmetic surgery. Although the Web sites of professional organizations might be preferred over commercial sites, you should also be aware that one of the roles of these organizations is to serve as an advocate for their members, and thus their Web sites are used to publicize cosmetic surgery and to guide you to the offices of their cosmetic surgeon members.

It makes sense to check out some of these sites initially to familiarize yourself with the procedures and terminology before seeking further information from an individual physician's site, or even before contacting a local cosmetic surgeon that you think you might like to do your surgery. The more information you find before selecting a physician, the better, as you will be able to evaluate what a physician posts on his or her Web site and

Internet Guide to Cosmetic Surgery for Men
© 2006 by The Haworth Press, Inc. All rights reserved.
doi:10.1300/5854_05

you will be better able to ask questions of the physician when you meet and talk with him or her about your potential surgery.

This chapter is organized into three primary sections. First is a group of sites that I consider "feature sites" which provide general information. These are primarily the sites of the membership organizations of physicians who perform cosmetic surgery, including the American Society of Plastic Surgeons. These sites are top-rated locations that feature a variety of procedures. They offer basic information about many cosmetic procedures; a few focus on one area of the body (e.g., the eye).

The second section consists of commercial sites that offer basic information about a variety of cosmetic procedures. Commercial sites make up the majority of the hundreds of thousands of sites about cosmetic surgery you will find on the Internet. Although many of the commercial sites on the Internet are the sites of individual doctors or groups of doctors, a few sites provide general cosmetic surgery information. Several are listed as examples.

The third section consists of a relatively small listing of sites that are directed specifically to men seeking cosmetic surgery information. One is a specific page from the American Society of Plastic Surgeons, and another is a site in the process of being launched. By the time this book is published I would anticipate many more sites of this type to have become available on the Internet.

In addition to the sites listed in this chapter, you are encouraged to begin your search with the appropriate sections in the two megasites that were listed in Chapter 2:

Ask NOAH About: Plastic and Cosmetic Surgery
<http://www.noah-health.org/English/procedures/plastic.html>

MedlinePlus—Plastic & Cosmetic Surgery
<http://www.nlm.nih.gov/medlineplus/plasticandcosmeticsurgery.html>

GENERAL SITES (.ORG) ON COSMETIC SURGERY PROCEDURES

American Academy of Cosmetic Surgery
<http://www.cosmeticsurgery.org>

The American Academy of Cosmetic Surgery (AACS) represents surgeons in many medical and surgical disciplines, all involved with cosmetic surgery. This site (see Figure 4.1) contains information for member surgeons, patients, and the media. Mouse over "Patient Information" and select "Surgeon Finder," "How to Choose a Surgeon," "Learn About a Procedure," "Patient FAQs," and more. At the time of evaluation, the site included patient information for nearly thirty procedures. The physician locator can be searched by doctor's last name, city, state, country, and/or procedure.

American Academy of Dermatology
<http://www.aad.org>

The American Academy of Dermatology (AAD) is "dedicated to achieving the highest quality of dermatologic care for everyone." The AAD, with

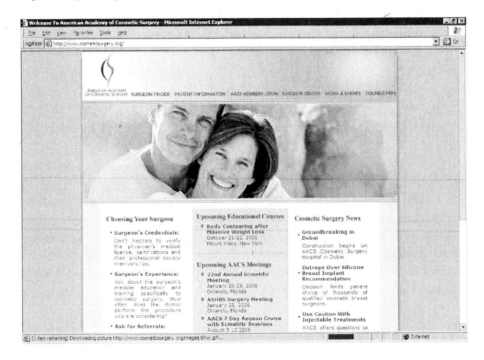

FIGURE 4.1. American Academy of Cosmetic Surgery Home Page
<http://www.cosmeticsurgery.org>
Reprinted with permission of American Academy of Cosmetic Surgery.

a membership of over 13,700, "is the largest, most influential and most representative of all dermatologic associations." Its Web site has information for both members and patients.

To access patient information about cosmetic surgery, under "Public Resource Center" select "Pamphlets." Pamphlets cover everything from dermatologic conditions to cosmetic surgery. Additional useful information for patients can be found in "News Room" under "News Releases."

Selecting "Find a Dermatologist" from the top bar of any page links you to a membership list of 13,000 dermatologists in the United States and worldwide. This is searchable by doctor's name, specialty, country, state or province, city, or location within a radius of a zip code.

American Academy of Facial Plastic and Reconstructive Surgery
<http://www.aafprs.org>
<http://www.facial-plastic-surgery.org>

The American Academy of Facial Plastic and Reconstructive Surgery (AAFPRS) is a specialty society of the American Medical Association representing over 2,700 members worldwide. AAFPRS members are board certified surgeons who deal with facial, head, and neck surgery.

The AAFPRS Web site states, "Trust Your Face to a Facial Plastic Surgeon." From the main page (see Figure 4.2), in the "Patients" section, select "Procedures." From that page you can then select the "Virtual Exam Room" that allows you to highlight the part of the face that you want surgery on, and then you can get information on the procedure. Or, "Procedure Types" links you directly to information on cosmetic surgical procedures of the face that are online adaptations of the academy's patient brochures. On the left-hand side, "Before and After" shows a photo gallery of selected procedures; in the FAQs you will find a glossary that defines technical medical terms, plus some statistics are available.

The AAFPRS's "Physician Finder" can be selected from any page. It is a membership directory of U.S. and Canadian facial plastic surgeons, and can be searched by state or province, city, zip code, or physician's name.

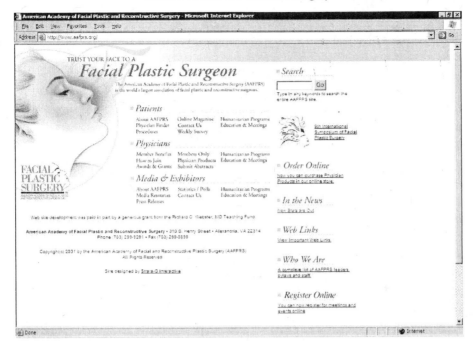

FIGURE 4.2. American Academy of Facial Plastic and Reconstructive Surgery Home Page
<http://www.aafprs.org>
Reprinted with permission of American Academy of Facial Plastic and Reconstructive Surgery.

American Society for Aesthetic Plastic Surgery
<http://www.surgery.org>

The American Society for Aesthetic Plastic Surgery (ASAPS) says that it is "the leading organization of plastic surgeons certified by the American Board of Plastic Surgery who specialize in cosmetic surgery of the face and body." Founded in 1967, it has approximately 2,100 members in the United States and Canada, as well as members in other countries. The ASAPS's site (see Figure 4.3) is a public information site providing cosmetic plastic surgery information; a section of the site is reserved for ASAPS members. Five major sections of the site guide potential patients to quality information.

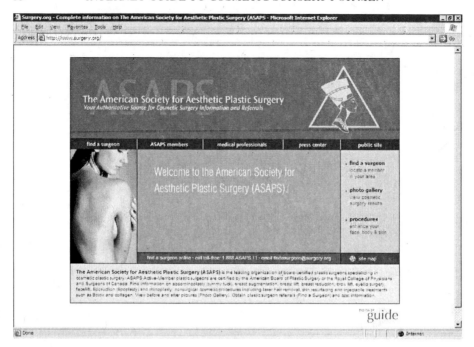

FIGURE 4.3. American Society of Aesthetic Plastic Surgery Home Page
<http://www.surgery.org>
Reprinted with permission of American Society of Aesthetic Plastic Surgery.

Selecting "Medical Professionals" from the main page guides you to information about the society, including its mission and qualifications for membership in ASAPS. Under "Public Site," select "Procedures" to go to a page of over twenty procedures, from which you can select the procedure(s) that interest you. Several of the topics are available in Spanish.

"Find a Surgeon" is one of the better doctor locators. You can locate a surgeon by name and/or city/state; by distances up to fifty miles from your zip code; or in locations outside the United States. The list of members is extensive.

This site has excellent information about cosmetic surgical procedures and is one of the main sites that make statistics available. Statistics can be accessed from the main page by selecting "Press Center" and then "Statistics" (available for every year from 1997 thru 2004, at the time of this review). This is certainly a location that you should check out for both background information and selecting a physician.

American Society for Dermatologic Surgery
<http://www.asds.net>

The American Society for Dermatologic Surgery was founded "to promote excellence in the subspecialty of dermatologic surgery and to foster the highest standards of patient care." This is a membership organization of board-certified dermatologists. The ASDS site (see Figure 4.4) has both a "members only" section and information for prospective patients. If you mouse over "Patients," you can then choose links to "Skin Care Corner," "Dermatologic Surgical Procedures," "Fact Sheets," "Before and After Photos," and more.

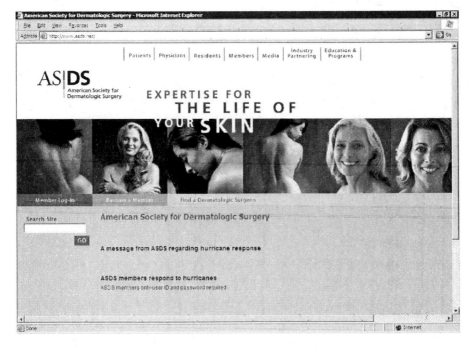

FIGURE 4.4. American Society for Dermatologic Surgery Home Page
<http://www.asds.net>
Reprinted with permission of American Society for Dermatologic Surgery.

Select "Fact Sheets" to link to information on over twenty-five specific procedures ("Dermatologic Surgical Procedures" contains definitions only). This site features everything from treatments on aging skin, spider veins and warts to hair restoration. Although you may think of this site for "skin only" surgery, you should know that liposuction, a body contouring procedure, was developed by dermatologic surgeons, and the ASDS site contains extensive information about this procedure. Specific pages from this site will be featured later under individual procedures.

"Find a Dermatologic Surgeon" can be selected from most pages. It is searchable by state or country and procedure, or by last name.

American Society of Ophthalmic Plastic and Reconstructive Surgery
\<http://www.asoprs.org\>

The American Society of Ophthalmic Plastic and Reconstructive Surgery (ASOPRS) is a membership organization of ophthalmologists who are certified by the American Board of Ophthalmology and have additional training and experience in plastic surgery of the "eyes and their surrounding structures," and have passed a specialized examination. There are "over 500 national and international members" of the society.

The ASOPRS Web site includes basic information about cosmetic surgery of the eyelids; this is accessed by mousing over "Society" and selecting "Patient Information." A "Membership Directory" can be selected from the menu bar. This directory is searchable by name, city, and state within the United States, and a small number of countries.

American Society of Plastic Surgeons
\<http://www.plasticsurgery.org\>

The American Society of Plastic Surgeons (ASPS) was founded in 1931. It is the "largest plastic surgery specialty organization in the world." Members of ASPS are board certified by either the American Board of Plastic Surgery or the Royal College of Physicians and Surgeons of Canada. "The mission of ASPS is to advance quality care to plastic surgery patients by encouraging high standards of training, ethics, physician practice and research in plastic surgery." The importance of board certification is discussed in Chapter 3.

The ASPS Web site (see Figure 4.5) provides public education about cosmetic and reconstructive plastic surgery, along with information specific to members of ASPS (password protected for members). The most prominent links on the page are "Find a Plastic Surgeon," "Learn about Procedures," and "News Room," but you should check out all of the links. The site is crammed with everything from statistics about the number of procedures performed by ASPS members (statistics are by year, age, sex, race, etc.) to information about qualifications required of board-certified surgeons and how to select a physician.

Select "Procedures" to get to "Learn About Procedures," and then select "Cosmetic Procedures" to get to "Cosmetic Plastic Surgery Procedures at a Glance," which gives general information about most cosmetic surgery

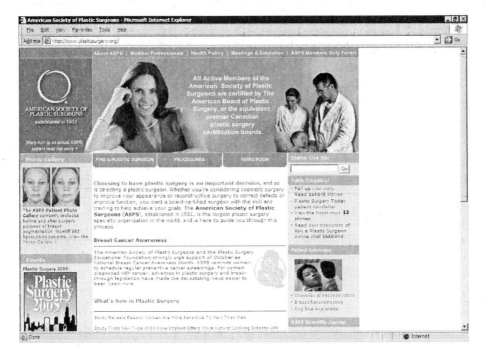

FIGURE 4.5. American Society of Plastic Surgeons Home Page
<http://www.plasticsurgery.org>

procedures. This overview of procedures includes a brief definition of the procedure (including the popular name of the procedure, e.g., abdominoplasty is a "tummy tuck"); length of time to perform the procedure; anesthesia used; whether it's an inpatient or outpatient procedure; risks involved; and recovery time. From this page, you can link to more detailed information about nearly twenty procedures. One of the selections is "Indications for Men"; this page is discussed in detail on p. 49 in this chapter. "Male Breast Reduction" is included in "Reconstructive Procedures" rather than "Cosmetic Procedures."

Selecting "Find a Plastic Surgeon" links you to the "Plastic Surgeon Referral Service." "All of the surgeons listed through the service are ASPS members who are board-certified by the American Board of Plastic Surgery and/or the Royal College of Physicians and Surgeons of Canada." This directory is searchable by the doctor's last name, procedure, address, city and state, or distance from a zip code. This plastic surgeon locator is the most comprehensive listing available on the Internet and recommended as the first place for you to begin locating a qualified surgeon in your area.

From the "News Room" on the main page, you can link to pages with official ASPS "Press Releases" and "Statistics." A photo gallery is also available. This site has a "site search" feature and many links both in the upper right-hand corner of the page, and along the left-hand side. This site is highly recommended as one of the best places to check for information.

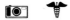

GENERAL SITES (.COM) ON COSMETIC SURGERY PROCEDURES

Cosmetic Surgery FYI
<http://www.cosmeticsurgeryfyi.com>

Cosmetic Surgery FYI, developed by Einstein Medical, Inc., is primarily a cosmetic surgeon locator site; however, it contains extensive information about numerous cosmetic surgery procedures including: liposuction, abdominoplasty, rhinoplasty, hair transplantation, facelifts, and Botox injections. The list of cosmetic surgeons on this site is not extensive, but information about a wide variety of cosmetic procedures makes it a valuable resource. This is the "parent" site of a group of FYI sites about specific types of cosmetic surgery, several of which will be listed in later chapters by the surgical procedure.

Facial Plastic Surgery Network
<http://www.facialplasticsurgery.net>

"The Facial Plastic Surgery Network is dedicated to helping you obtain solutions to your facial aesthetic concerns." This site is produced by Enhancement Media, a company that has a group of related sites on many cosmetic surgery topics. The site is easy to navigate, with links at the top of the home page to "Facial Procedures," "Choosing a Surgeon," "Procedure FAQ," "Anesthesia Information," a photo gallery, financing information, chat groups and discussion forums, and more (see Figure 4.6). The key

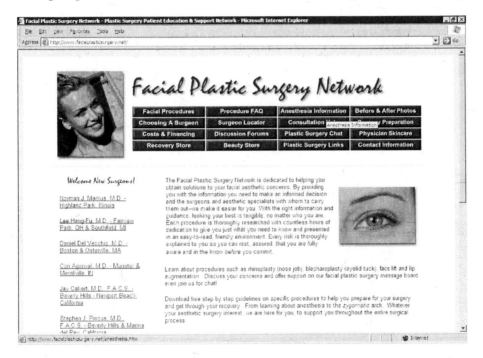

FIGURE 4.6. Facial Plastic Surgery Network Home Page
<http://www.facialplasticsurgery.net>
Reprinted with permission of Enhancement Media.

page is "Facial Procedures," which has links to an extensive list of procedures, divided by type of procedure (e.g., skin). Information is similar to the site **Yes They're Fake!** that is also produced by the same company, just without the candid commentary. The information about each procedure is extensive, covering everything from the procedure itself to risks and complications. Especially useful is a link to a page about how to evaluate your physician's credentials. This site, and the other sites by Enhancement Media, are all interlinked and share chat groups and discussion forums. Chat groups and the discussion forums are useful because you can have online discussions about cosmetic procedures with others who have had, or are contemplating, the same procedure.

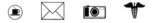

iEnhance
<http://www.ienhance.com>

iEnhance indicates that its "mission is to help people attain a more attractive body and image." The iEnhance site (see Figure 4.7) serves primarily as a locator service of "qualified plastic surgeons, cosmetic surgeons, dermatologists, cosmetic dentists and vision correction specialists." It indicates that all physicians listed are board certified by the American Board of Plastic Surgery. The list of surgeons can be accessed by specialty, state or country, or doctor's last name. The site includes information on specific procedures (select "Procedures," then "Plastic Surgery" or "Facial Plastic Surgery" to bring up an extensive list). From the home page, you can also select "Plastic Surgery," "Facial Plastic Surgery," "Dermatology," "Cosmetic Dentistry," or "Vision," to go to these specialty pages where you will find featured articles and links to surgical procedures and more. The site also includes a photo gallery, message board, and financing information for patients.

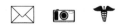

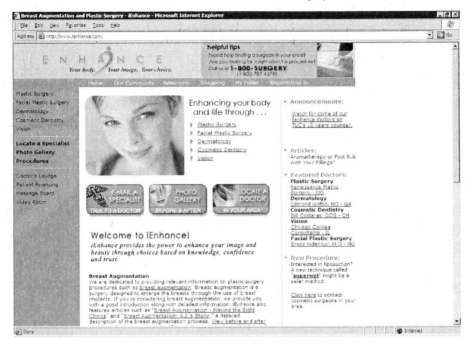

FIGURE 4.7. iEnhance Home Page
<http://www.ienhance.com>
Reprinted with permission of iEnhance.com.

Medem
<http://www.medem.com>

The Medem Network, designed to facilitate physician-patient communication, maintains a "full range of patient education information from . . . partner societies and other trusted sources." The site includes information for physicians, patients, and industries (e.g., health plans and systems). Select "For Patients" from the home page, then "Browse Topics." Under "Therapies and Health Strategies," select "Plastic Surgery/Cosmetic and Reconstructive Procedures." Links from this page go to Insurance Issues, Plastic Surgery Basics, Procedures of the Breast, Liposuction, Other Cosmetic Procedures, Statistics, among other topics. The majority of the material available from Medem was produced by organizations such as the

American Society of Plastic Surgeons and the American Academy of Facial, Plastic and Reconstructive Surgery.

Yes They're Fake!
<http://www.yestheyrefake.net>

Yes They're Fake! is a refreshingly candid (see Figure 4.8) site that is fun to read. The actual content (surgical procedure, risks, complications, anesthesia, etc.) duplicates what can be found on the **Facial Plastic Surgery Network <http://www.facialplasticsurgery.net>** (listed previously). However, it's the personal commentary that makes this site so unique and interesting. This site has "attitude."

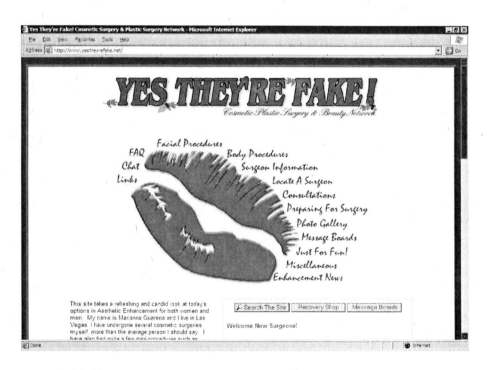

FIGURE 4.8. Yes They're Fake! Home Page
<http://www.yestheyrefake.net>
Reprinted with permission of Enhancement Media.

GENERAL SITES ON COSMETIC SURGERY FOR MEN

About.com—Men's Health—Cosmetic Surgery and Men
\<http://menshealth.about.com/od/cosmeticsurgery/\>

The Men's Health section on about.com includes a page on Cosmetic Surgery and Men. From this page you can link to articles/resources on topics that range from pectoral implants, gynecomastia, and hair transplantation to "Nips & Tucks for Men."

American Society of Plastic Surgeons—Plastic Surgery Indications for Men
\<http://www.plasticsurgery.org/public_education/procedures/Plastic SurgeryForMen.cfm\>

The ASPS site is listed earlier in the chapter. This page was developed specifically for men who are considering cosmetic surgery (see Figure 4.9). Go directly to the URL, or select from the list of cosmetic procedures. The page discusses planning the surgery and what the surgeon should discuss with you, along with some specific issues related to men that may influence the surgery (e.g., men have a richer blood supply in the face; shaving needs to be postponed with some skin procedures; and skin elasticity differs between men and women).

Bermant Plastic and Cosmetic Surgery—Male Plastic Surgery
\<http://www.plasticsurgery4u.com/male_plastic_surgery.index.html\>

This site is provided by Dr. Michael Bermant, a board certified physician in plastic surgery, who practices near Richmond, Virginia. The site is not well organized, but it contains a wealth of information. Go directly to the URL, or, from the main page you can select "Male Plastic & Cosmetic Surgery" from the bar on the right-hand side. Topics include male chest sculpture (gynecomastia); male liposuction, tummy tuck and body contouring; and more. An extensive photo gallery of male cosmetic surgery patients is available. The site subscribes to the HONcode principles.

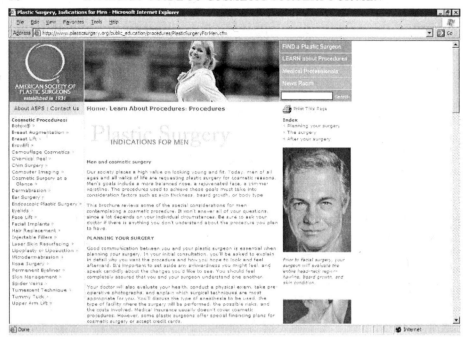

FIGURE 4.9. American Society of Plastic Surgeons—Plastic Surgery Indications
for Men
<http://www.plasticsurgery.org/public_education/procedures/PlasticSurgeryForMen.cfm>
©2004 American Society of Plastic Surgeons. All rights reserved. Learn more at
<www.plasticsurgery.org>.

Institute of Cosmetic Surgery—Male Cosmetic Surgery
<http://www.cosmeticscanada.com/male-cosmetic-surgery.html>

The Institute of Cosmetic Surgery is the cosmetic surgery practice site of
Dr. L. Tarshis. This page gives basic information about reasons why men
elect to have cosmetic surgery and links to descriptions of popular procedures. It is an example of a physician's site with information specific to men.

Plastic Surgery 4 Men
<http://www.surgery4men.com>

Plastic Surgery 4 Men is "dedicated to helping men obtain solutions to
their every aesthetic concern." This site bills itself as "a patient education
and support network for males only." The site is still under construction (see

Figure 4.10). It is being developed by Enhancement Media, which also puts up a number of cosmetic surgery sites including **Yes They're Fake!** Tabs indicate a similar approach to information as at their other sites—e.g., facial procedures, body procedures, anesthesia choices, costs, surgeon information, and more, only with a focus on men. The message board (a discussion forum) was functional in fall 2005. This site promises to be a major resource for men considering cosmetic surgery when it is completed.

NEXT: INTERNET SITES FOR SPECIFIC COSMETIC SURGERY PROCEDURES

The Web sites in this chapter will be listed many times in the remaining chapters of this book, but you will be guided to specific cosmetic proce-

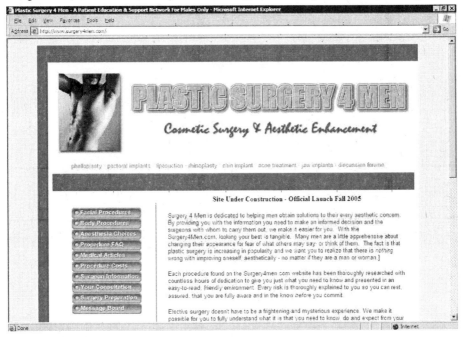

FIGURE 4.10. Plastic Surgery 4 Men
<http://www.surgery4men.com>
Reprinted with permission of Enhancement Media.

dures within each Web site. One of your choices is to use these sites "in general"—to go directly to whichever site you have chosen (e.g., American Society of Plastic Surgeons or the American Academy of Facial Plastic and Reconstructive Surgery), and simply explore the many procedures and information located on each site. Or, you can go directly to the specific cosmetic surgery procedure in which you are interested by using the direct links in the remainder of this book. By dividing chapters into logical groupings by body site, you should easily find the procedure(s) that you are interested in. This will also allow you to browse for related procedures. Cross-references guide you within chapters, and the index can also be used to locate the cosmetic procedure that you are considering.

Chapter 5

Body Contouring

This chapter covers body contouring procedures, or reshaping of the body. Liposuction was the top cosmetic surgery reported for men in 2004 by the American Society for Aesthetic Plastic Surgery, and the fourth most popular surgical procedure for men in 2004 by the American Society of Plastic Surgeons. Liposuction (lipoplasty) is one of the primary surgical procedures covered in this chapter; also included are surgeries such as tummy tucks (abdominoplasty), buttock augmentation, and calf implants. Please follow cross-references, which lead to other sections in this chapter or to other chapters. In general, the "common" name rather than the technical name is used for a procedure.

Male breast reduction, performed for the treatment of gynecomastia, could also be considered body contouring. Because this surgery is done exclusively in men, it has been included in a chapter devoted to procedures for men (see Chapter 6, "Cosmetic Procedures Specific to Men").

BODY CONTOURING—GENERAL

Bermant Plastic and Cosmetic Surgery
<http://www.plasticsurgery4u.com>

This is the site of Dr. Michael Bermant, a board-certified physician in plastic surgery, who practices near Richmond, Virginia. The site lacks organization but contains a wealth of information. Near the top of the page is "Body Plastic Surgery Sculpture," where you will find links to information

Internet Guide to Cosmetic Surgery for Men
© 2006 by The Haworth Press, Inc. All rights reserved.
doi:10.1300/5854_06

on liposuction, tummy tuck, and more. The "Site Search" feature is also useful. The site subscribes to the HONcode principles.

Yes They're Fake!—Body Enhancement
<http://www.yestheyrefake.net/body_plastic_surgery.html>

This site was created by a patient who has undergone cosmetic surgery. The "Body Enhancement" page is an alphabetic list of approximately thirty cosmetic procedures, many of which are also listed individually in this chapter and in Chapter 6.

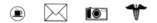

ABDOMINAL LIPOSCULPTURE (LIPOSUCTION)

See also LIPOSUCTION; TUMMY TUCK (ABDOMINOPLASTY).
Abdominal liposuction removes fat from the abdomen and reshapes the abdominal area.

iEnhance—Abdominal Liposculpture
<http://www.ienhance.com/procedure/default.asp>

From the "List of Procedures," select "Plastic Surgery," then under "Abdomen" select "Abdominal Liposculpture (Liposuction)." This page (see Figure 5.1) includes basic information such as patient selection, surgical procedure, risks, and postsurgical recovery.

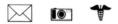

ARM LIFT (BRACHIOPLASTY)/ARM LIPOSUCTION/UPPER ARM LIFT

Brachioplasty, also called upper arm lift, is the surgical reduction of the upper arm to remove loose, hanging skin that may occur due to aging or weight loss. With arm liposuction, fat is first suctioned out of the arm; follow-up surgery may be required to remove excess skin.

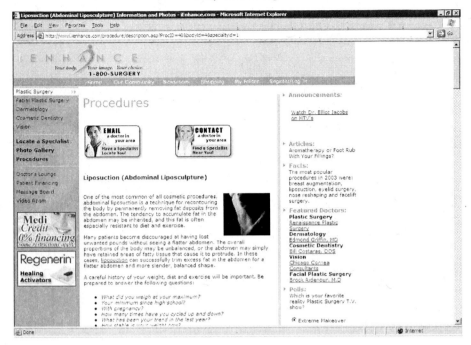

FIGURE 5.1. iEnhance—Abdominal Liposculpture
<http://www.ienhance.com/procedure/description.asp?ProcID=40andbodyid=4andsp
ecialtyid=1>
Reprinted with permission of iEnhance.com.

2004 statistics:

ASAPS: 17,052 (832 in men)
ASPS: 9,955 (398 in men)

American Academy of Cosmetic Surgery—Upper Arm Lift
<http://www.cosmeticsurgery.org/Patients/upperarmlift.asp>

This provides a brief description of the procedure, including post-surgery information. Scarring is a trade-off with the procedure.

American Society of Plastic Surgeons—Brachioplasty
<http://www.plasticsurgery.org/public_education/procedures/
Brachioplasty.cfm>

This page provides a brief description of the procedure.

Columbia University Department of Surgery—Upper Arm Lift
<http://www.columbiasurgery.org/divisions/plastic/cp_arm.html>

This page from Columbia University describes the upper arm lift procedure, how it's done, and provides before and after surgery information.

eMedicine—Liposuction, Upper Arms
<http://www.emedicine.com/plastic/topic31.htm>

This article by Dr. JoAnne Lopes describes liposuction in the upper
arms. It's a bit technical, covering the procedure and methods of assessing
patients as candidates for upper arm liposuction.

iEnhance—Arm Liposuction
<http://www.ienhance.com/procedure/default.asp>

From the "List of Procedures," select "Plastic Surgery" and then, under
"Arms," select "Arm Liposuction" and/or "Arm Lifts/Brachioplasty." Gives
basic information about the procedure, risks, what to expect post-surgery,
questions to ask your surgeon, and costs.

BELT LIPECTOMY

See LOWER BODY LIFT.

BODY LIFT

See LOWER BODY LIFT.

BUTTOCK AUGMENTATION/IMPLANT

Buttock augmentation is a surgical procedure for reshaping and increasing the size of the buttocks, either to create a balanced look, or to simply enlarge the buttock area. This is accomplished with either an implant (silicone) or through micro fat grafting.

2004 statistics:

ASAPS: 2,141   (58 in men)

American Academy of Cosmetic Surgery—Buttock Implants
<http://www.cosmeticsurgery.org/Patients/buttockimplants.asp>

The procedure is briefly described.

Yes They're Fake!—Buttock Augmentation
<http://www.yestheyrefake.net/buttock_augmentation.htm>

The page describes the surgery and types of augmentation (implants versus micro fat grafting), recovery (including pre-op and post-op instructions), risks and complications, questions to ask, and more.

BUTTOCK LIFT/LIPOSCULPTURE/LIPOSUCTION

Buttock liposuction removes fat from the buttocks and reshapes the buttock area.

2004 statistics:

ASAPS: 5,960   (520 in men)
ASPS: 3,496   (210 in men)

eMedicine—Body Contouring, Buttocks Surgery
\<http://www.emedicine.com/plastic/topic15.htm\>

This article on buttock surgery, by Dr. Neal R. Reisman, discusses contouring of the buttocks area, including implants; however, the majority of the article is about reduction of the buttocks.

iEnhance—Buttock Liposculpture/Liposuction
\<http://www.ienhance.com/procedure/default.asp\>

From the "List of Procedures," select "Plastic Surgery" and then, under "Buttocks/Groin," select "Buttock Liposculpture/Liposuction." The page gives basic information about the procedure, best candidates, risks, what to expect postsurgery, questions to ask your surgeon, and costs.

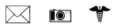

CALF AUGMENTATION/IMPLANTS

Calf augmentation reshapes the lower legs. In the procedure, an implant (such as silicone) is inserted into the leg to give it more shape and definition.

2004 statistics:

ASAPS: 226   (127 were men)

American Academy of Cosmetic Surgery—Calf Implants
\<http://www.cosmeticsurgery.org/Patients/calflift.asp\>

Calf enlargement is described, including the implant material. This procedure is often used by body builders.

iEnhance—Calf Implants
<http://www.ienhance.com/procedure/default.asp>

From the "List of Procedures," select "Plastic Surgery" and then, under "Legs," select "Calf Implant." This page gives basic information about the procedure, risks, what to expect postsurgery, questions to ask your surgeon, and costs.

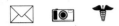

Yes They're Fake!—Calf Augmentation
<http://www.yestheyrefake.net/calf_augmentation_implants.htm>

Included in this page is a description of the surgery and types of augmentation (implants versus micro fat grafting), recovery (including pre-op and post-op instructions), risks and complications, questions to ask, and more.

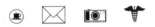

FLANKOPLASTY

See LOWER BODY LIFT.

LIPOSUCTION

According to the American Society for Aesthetic Plastic Surgery, liposuction was the number one elective cosmetic surgical procedure for men in the United States in 2004; the American Society of Plastic Surgeons ranks it as the fourth most popular surgical procedure for men. Liposuction is defined by the ASPS as "a procedure that can help sculpt the body by removing unwanted fat from specific areas, including the abdomen, hips, buttocks, thighs, upper arms, chin, cheeks and neck."[1] By removing fat, weight loss occurs, but liposuction should not be considered solely as a weight loss method. The best candidates for liposuction keep their bodies fit; they exercise and eat the right foods, but may have stubborn areas of fat that just will not come off despite proper diet and exercise. Several methods of liposuction can be used, but the most common is tumescent liposuction, in which fluid containing lidocaine (an anesthetic) is injected into the area where fat is to be removed. This provides some local anesthesia and makes it easier for the cannula, a small tube used in this procedure, to break up fat and remove it.

Liposuction information is easily found on the Internet; in fact, a recent Google search brought up about 1,350,000 "hits." Sites that come up first from a general search using an Internet browser are not always the best sites. Following are some recommended sites that include both professional and reviewed sites, along with a representative selection of commercial sites.

2004 statistics:

ASAPS: 478,251   (61,638 in men)
ASPS: 324,891   (32,489 in men)

American Academy of Cosmetic Surgery—Liposuction
\<http://www.cosmeticsurgery.org/Patients/liposuction.asp\>

This site provides a brief description of liposuction.

American Academy of Dermatology—Tumescent Liposuction
\<http://www.aad.org/public/Publications/pamphlets/Liposuction.htm\>

This AAD online pamphlet describes liposuction, focusing specifically on tumescent liposuction. The pamphlet covers the procedure and its benefits, indications for the surgery, and why a patient would choose a dermatologic surgeon for this procedure. Postsurgery and safety information are included. Also of interest, but more technical, is the page "Guidelines of Care for Liposuction" <http://www.aad.org/professionals/guidelines/Liposuction.htm>, intended for the dermatology professional.

American Society for Aesthetic Plastic Surgery—Liposuction (Lipoplasty)
\<http://www.surgery.org/public/procedures-lipoplasty.php\>

The format for this page requires you to select "next" to get to all of the information about liposuction. This is an excellent place to begin your search. It contains everything from a description of various liposuction procedures to before and after surgery and potential complications. Also included are illustrations, plus a photo gallery, and an extensive "Find a Surgeon" feature. This page is also available in Spanish.

American Society for Dermatologic Surgery
\<http://www.asds.net/Patients/FactSheets/patients-Fact_Sheet-liposuction.html\>
\<http://www.asds.net/Patients/FactSheets/patients-Fact_Sheet-skinny_on_lipo.html\>

The ASDS site features liposuction information in several sections of its Web page. The focus is on tumescent liposuction. "The Skinny on Liposuction" and the fact sheet on "Liposuction" (see Figure 5.2) contain unique but overlapping information promoting liposuction. The two pages cover everything from benefits and complications to misconceptions and new technologies/advances. The site claims that approximately one-third of all liposuction procedures in the United States are performed by dermatologic surgeons. "Find a Dermatologic Surgeon" locates a physician near you.

American Society of Plastic Surgeons—Lipoplasty (Liposuction)
\<http://www.plasticsurgery.org/public_education/procedures/Lipoplasty.cfm\>

The ASPS public information page on liposuction includes a surgery description, best candidates for surgery, anesthesia information, technique variations, risks, postsurgical recovery, and before/after illustrations. This is one of the more extensive pages about liposuction and a top choice for beginning your search for information. This page is available

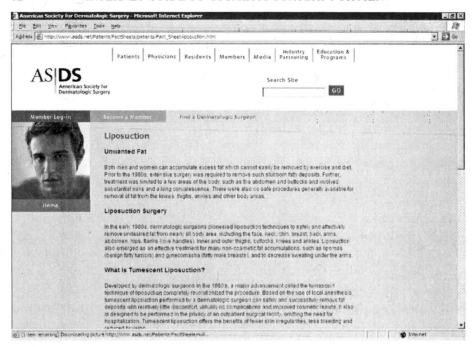

FIGURE 5.2. American Society for Dermatologic Surgery—Liposuction
<http://www.asds.net/Patients/FactSheets/patients-Fact_Sheet-liposuction.html>
Reprinted with permission of American Society for Dermatologic Surgery.

in Spanish (choose Spanish from Procedures page or go directly to
<http://www.plasticsurgery.org/public_education/procedures/Liposuccion.
cfm>). You should also check out the description of the tumescent technique at <http://www.plasticsurgery.org/public_education/procedures/
LiposuctionTumescentTechnique.cfm>.

iEnhance.com
<http://www.ienhance.com>

This site separates its information about liposuction into specific areas
of the body. Look elsewhere in this chapter under ABDOMINAL LIPO-

SCULPTURE (LIPOSUCTION); ARM LIPOSUCTION; BUTTOCK LIPOSCULP-TURE/LIPOSUCTION; and THIGH LIPOSCULPTURE; and in Chapter 7, "Cosmetic Surgery of the Face, Head, and Neck," under NECK LIFT/NECK LIPOSUCTION.

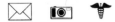

Lipoinfo.com
<http://www.lipoinfo.com>

This is the site of Dr. Paul Weber of Ft. Lauderdale, Florida. It claims to be "the most comprehensive liposuction information site on the Internet," and very well may be. Information includes everything from the history of liposuction, definitions, and anatomy to details on the types of liposuction, procedures, anaesthesia, side effects, and before-and-after pictures. Dr. Weber's extensive curriculum vitae includes board certification in dermatology, specialized fellowship in dermatologic surgery, patented medical instruments, and a long list of publications. The site provides information for potential patients who evidently travel to Florida from throughout the United States and the world to have liposuction performed by Dr. Weber, so the site definitely has a commercial intent. However, Dr. Weber's presentation about liposuction, its proper use, and complications offers a unique perspective that is worth reading. The style is unique and offers information not available on other sites. Information in Spanish is available here, also.

Liposuction 4 You
<http://www.liposuction4you.com>

This site is produced by Enhancement Media, a company that has a group of sites on many cosmetic surgery topics. The site is easy to navigate (see Figure 5.3), with links to "Your Anatomy," "Learn About Liposuction," "Surgery Information," "Road to Recovery," selecting a surgeon, costs and financing, professional organizations worldwide, and more. Within each page are links to fairly extensive information; for example, the surgical procedure page contains topics such as: "How much fat can be safely removed in one procedure?" and "Does fat 'grow

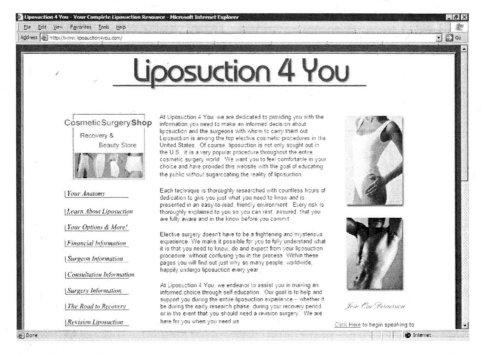

FIGURE 5.3. Liposuction 4 You
<http://www.liposuction4you.com>
Reprinted with permission of Enhancement Media.

back'?" Within "Plastic Surgeon Information" are links to help you research your surgeon and how to select a good surgeon. "Just for Fun" includes a chat room.

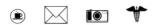

Liposuction Consumer Guide
<http://www.liposuction-consumer-guide.com>

The site includes basic information on liposuction, for example, types of procedures, benefits, risks, and questions to ask your surgeon. The site features a locator service to find a liposuction surgeon in your local area, but the list is not extensive.

LiposuctionFYI.com
<http://www.liposuctionfyi.com/index.html>

This site is a special section of the CosmeticSurgeryFYI.com site that provides extensive information about the liposuction surgical procedure, whether you are a candidate for the procedure, risks, options available, and FAQs. It contains links to before/after photos. The commercial aspect is evident with a link to the Liposuction DocShop on each page, plus financing information.

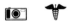

MayoClinic.com—Liposuction: Considerations About Body
Sculpting
<http://www.mayoclinic.com>

Go to the general Mayo Clinic site <http://www.mayoclinic.com> and do a site search for "liposuction." This page gives an honest appraisal of what liposuction can and cannot do, questions to ask your surgeon, techniques of liposuction (tumescent and ultrasonic), preparing for liposuction, postsurgery information, and risks of the procedure.

U.S. Food and Drug Administration. Center for Devices
and Radiological Health—Liposuction Information
<http://www.fda.gov/cdrh/liposuction>

The Food and Drug Administration (FDA) regulates drugs (e.g., anesthetics) and medical devices, including equipment used to perform liposuction. The FDA site (see Figure 5.4) has basic information about liposuction and who performs the procedure, risks and complications, and "What can I expect?" before, during, and after the surgery. Alternatives to liposuction are given and Information about where to report a problem can be

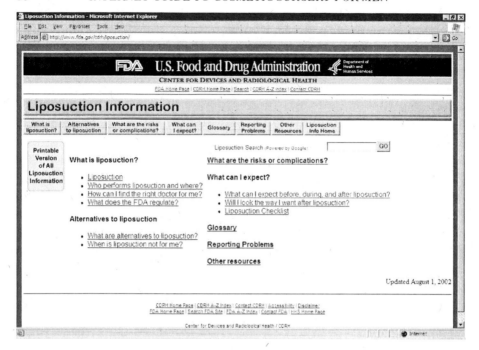

FIGURE 5.4. U.S. FDA—Liposuction Information
<http://www.fda.gov/cdrh/liposuction>

found here. Anyone considering liposuction should go to this site to read about the risks/complications. Click "Printable Version of All Liposuction Information" or go directly to <http://www.fda.gov/cdrh/liposuction/complete.html> to get a printable version of all liposuction pages linked to this FDA page. This should be required reading for anyone considering liposuction.

Yes They're Fake!—Liposuction
<http://www.yestheyrefake.net/liposuction.htm>

The page describes the surgery, indications and contraindications for liposuction, risks and complications, and more. You are referred to a related site—**Liposuction 4 You <http://www.liposuction4you.com>** (see separate listing).

LOWER BODY LIFT

Terminology varies with this procedure, but it was easiest to place body lifts, lower body lifts, belt lipectomy, and flankoplasty under one listing. Belt lipectomy is described as doing a "facelift" on the entire torso. It is an extensive procedure and not offered at many locations; two of the sites originate with the University of Iowa.

2004 statistics:

ASAPS: 15,094 (1,716 in men)
ASPS: 8,926 (1,250 in men)

eMedicine—Body Contouring, Flankoplasty and Thigh Lift
<http://www.emedicine.com/plastic/topic524.htm>

The article on this site by Bruce G. Freeman is referenced and linked from several other sites on the Internet. Included are several pictures, about half of which show this procedure in men.

University of Iowa Health Care—Belt Lipectomy
for Circumferential Truncal Excess
<http://www.uihealthcare.com/news/currents.vol3issue4/04belt.html>

Drs. Al Aly and Zlaitko Agnuelov author this brief news item on belt lipectomy, a procedure which involves removal of excess skin and fatty tissue that surrounds the trunk or body. "Belt lipectomy is indicated in three types of patients. The majority . . . are patients who have had a significant loss of weight due to gastric/intestinal bypass surgery. . . ." As more individuals undergo bariatric surgery, this operation will become more common. Dr. Aly has been quoted in the news and has published papers on this topic. The University of Iowa Health Care Web site has absorbed much of what was formerly the Virtual Hospital (discontinued January 1, 2006).

THIGH LIPOSUCTION (THIGHPLASTY)/THIGH LIFT

Thigh liposuction is the removal of fat to reshape the thigh; it can be done to remove fat deposits on both the inner and outer thigh area. Thigh lifts are frequently done in conjunction with a lower body lift.

2004 statistics:

ASAPS: 13,502   (728 in men)
ASPS: 8,123   (406 in men)

American Academy of Cosmetic Surgery—Thighlift
<http://www.cosmeticsurgery.org/Patients/thighlift.asp>

This site provides a brief description of the surgery, including anesthesia and postsurgery information.

iEnhance—Thigh Liposculpture
<http://www.ienhance.com/procedures/default.asp>

From the "List of Procedures," select "Plastic Surgery," then under "Legs" select "Thigh Liposculpture." This page includes basic information about thighplasty, from selection of patients and the surgical procedure through risks, postsurgery, and costs. A link to "Leg Lift" is incomplete and has photos only.

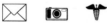

TUMMY TUCK (ABDOMINOPLASTY)

Tummy tuck (abdominoplasty) is a surgical procedure that removes fat and skin from the tummy area, while also tightening the abdominal muscles. Tummy tucks are often performed in conjunction with liposuction.

2004 statistics:

ASAPS: 150,987   (5,672 in men)
ASPS: 107,019   (4,281 in men)

American Academy of Cosmetic Surgery—Abdominoplasty (Tummy Tuck)
<http://www.cosmeticsurgery.org/Patients/abdominoplasty.asp>

The tummy tuck procedure is briefly described.

American Society for Aesthetic Plastic Surgery—Tummy Tuck
<http://www.surgery.org/public/procedures-tummytuck.php>

The ASAPS page on tummy tucks has basic information about who is a good candidate for the procedure, the surgery itself, risks, and what to expect after the procedure. This page is also available in Spanish.

American Society of Plastic Surgeons—Abdominoplasty (Tummy Tuck)
<http://www.plasticsurgery.org/public_education/procedures/ Abdominoplasty.cfm>

The ASPS public information page on tummy tucks includes a description of the surgery, best candidates, preparing for surgery, risks, postsurgical recovery, and before/after illustrations.

iEnhance—Abdominoplasty (Tummy Tuck)
<http://www.ienhance.com/procedure/default.asp>

From the "List of Procedures," select "Plastic Surgery," then under "Abdomen" select "Abdominoplasty (Tummy Tuck)." This page includes basic information about tummy tucks, from the selection of patients and the surgical procedure to the risks, postsurgery, and costs.

Tuck That Tummy!
<http://www.tuckthattummy.com>

This site is produced by Enhancement Media, a company that has a group of sites on cosmetic surgery topics. The site is easy to navigate, with links on the left-hand side that go to pages on "Your Anatomy," the surgical procedure, "Road to Recovery," selecting a surgeon, costs and financing, and more. Within each page are links to fairly extensive information; for example, the surgical procedure page includes topics such as: "Preparing yourself emotionally" and an extensive description of the procedure with diagrams. Within "Plastic Surgeon Information" are links to help you research your surgeon (medical license, certifications, malpractice, etc.) and how to select a surgeon. The photo gallery is located under "Miscellaneous Information."

 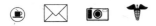

Tummy Tuck Resource
<http://www.tummy-tuck-resource.com>

This site bills itself as "a safety and resource site for abdominoplasty surgery." It includes photographs, risks, a description of the surgery, anesthesia, and what to expect following the procedure. "Find a Tummy Tuck Surgeon in Your Area," listed by state, appears on each page, but when you select a state and then your area within the state, only a form comes up to contact a doctor, without giving a doctor's name.

Yes They're Fake!—Abdominoplasty
<http://www.yestheyrefake.net/abdominoplasty.htm>

The page describes indications for the surgery and whether you are a good candidate for the types of procedures (types of incisions and endoscopic abdominoplasty to mini versus full abdominoplasty), risks and complications, and more.

UPPER ARM LIFT

See ARM LIFT (BRACHIOPLASTY)/ARM LIPOSUCTION/UPPER ARM LIFT.

NOTE

1. "Lipoplasty." American Society of Plastic Surgeons. Available: <http://www.plasticsurgery.org/public_education/procedures/Lipoplasty.cfm>.

Chapter 6

Cosmetic Procedures Specific to Men

This chapter includes information about locating Web sites on three procedures that are specific to men: gynecomastia, in which male breast reduction is performed; pectoral (or male chest) augmentation/implants; and phalloplasty, or penis enlargement/implants. Other procedures such as calf implants, which can be performed on both men and women, can be found in Chapter 5 "Body Contouring."

GYNECOMASTIA-MALE BREAST REDUCTION

Gynecomastia, or male breast enlargement, is actually more common than one might expect. Estimates show that up to 60 percent of males have gynecomastia. The most frequent cause of gynecomastia is hormonal changes, frequently at puberty. However, hormonal changes due to other body changes, tumors, prescription drugs, or hereditary factors can also cause gynecomastia. Depending on the extent of the breast enlargement, treatments might range from simple diet and exercise, to hormonal treatment or surgery. Sometimes, no matter how much you diet and exercise, you simply cannot reduce the size of your breasts and may wish to consider surgery.

A recent search on Google found over 721,000 sites for male breast reduction, and another 347,000 for gynecomastia—obviously too much to wade through to locate good information. The following selected sites focus on surgical treatment for gynecomastia.

Internet Guide to Cosmetic Surgery for Men
© 2006 by The Haworth Press, Inc. All rights reserved.
doi:10.1300/5854_07

73

2004 statistics:

ASAPS: 19,636 (all male)
ASPS: 13,963 (all male)

American Academy of Cosmetic Surgery—Gynecomastia
<http://www.cosmeticsurgery.org/Patients/gynecomastia.asp>

This Web page (see Figure 6.1) includes a brief description of the procedure, reasons why the procedure is performed, and postsurgical recovery.

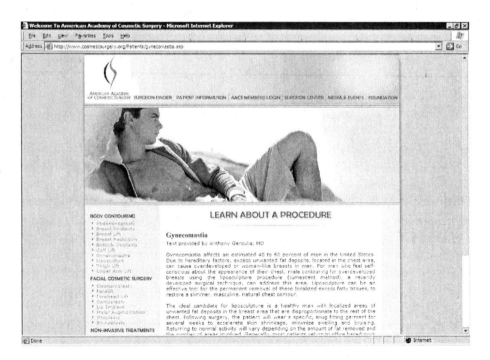

FIGURE 6.1. American Academy of Cosmetic Surgery—Gynecomastia
<http://www.cosmeticsurgery.org/Patients/gynecomastia.asp>
Reprinted with permission of American Academy of Cosmetic Surgery.

American Society for Aesthetic Plastic Surgery—Male Breast Reduction (Treatment of Gynecomastia)
<http://www.surgery.org/press/procedurefacts-malebreast.php>

This ASAPS page discusses the procedure for male breast reduction via liposuction and excision of excessive glandular tissue. Benefits and possible complications are listed. A before-and-after photo is available in the Liposuction photo gallery at <http://www.surgery.org/public/procedure photo.php/304>.

American Society of Plastic Surgeons—Gynecomastia (Male Breast Reduction)
<http://www.plasticsurgery.org/public_education/procedures/ Gynecomastia.cfm>

This ASPS page (see Figure 6.2) describes gynecomastia (it affects 40 to 60 percent of men), indicates who are the best candidates for surgery, describes the surgery (risks, planning, anesthesia, procedure, and postsurgery), and discusses expectations for your new look.

Bermant Plastic and Cosmetic Surgery—Gynecomastia
<http://www.plasticsurgery4u.com/procedure_folder/male_breast/ index.html>

This site is provided by Dr. Michael Bermant, a board certified physician in plastic surgery, who practices near Richmond, Virginia. Go directly to the URL, or scroll until you get to "Gynecomastia" and then link to information about male breast-reduction surgery. The site subscribes to the HONcode principles.

eMedicine—Gynecomastia
<http://www.emedicine.com/plastic/topic125.htm>

This fairly technical article by Dr. Fawzi Ali describes the medical condition of gynecomastia, including etiology, pathophysiology, and clinical pre-

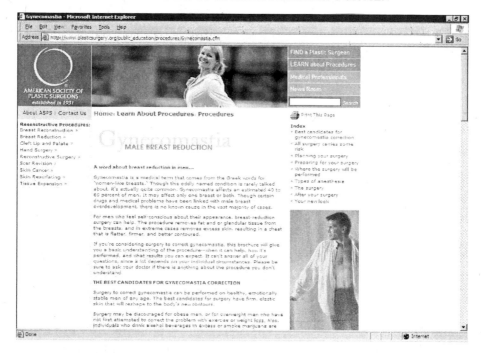

FIGURE 6.2. American Society of Plastic Surgeons—Gynecomastia (Male Breast
   Reduction)
<http://www.plasticsurgery.org/public_education/procedures/Gynecomastia.cfm>
©2004 American Society of Plastic Surgeons. All rights reserved. Learn more at
   <www.plasticsurgery.org>.

sentation, and then describes both the medical and surgical treatments for
the disorder. Surgery involves resection (subcutaneous mastectomy) and
liposuction-assisted mastectomy. Photos and diagrams are included. A second article on mastectomy <http://www.emedicine.com/med/topic934.htm>
focuses on causes, laboratory tests, and medical care.

iEnhance—Gynecomastia (Male Breast Reduction)
<http://www.ienhance.com/procedure/default.asp>

From the "List of Procedures" select "Plastic Surgery," then under "Breast"
select "Gynecomastia (Male Breast Reduction)." The page includes infor-

mation about the surgical consultation, the ideal candidate, questions to ask the doctor, the surgical procedure, risks, recovery, and results. Alternatives to surgery are listed, along with costs.

Pec Implants.com—Gynecomastia
<http://www.pecimplants.com/gynecomastia.html>

This site is provided by Dr. Smith, who specializes in cosmetic surgery involving muscle contouring. Although the information about gynecomastia is useful, the site is missing any information about Dr. Smith's qualifications—even where the practice is located, so inclusion here is not an endorsement.

Yes They're Fake!—Gynecomastia
<http://www.yestheyrefake.net/gynecomastia.htm>

This Web page (see Figure 6.3) describes what gynecomastia is, options for treatment, what to expect during a surgical consult, the surgery and how to prepare for it, along with the recovery and risks and complications.

PECTORAL (MALE CHEST) AUGMENTATION/IMPLANTS

Pectoral augmentation is a procedure done in men when the chest area needs to be enlarged. Often, this surgery is done for congenital defects such as spina bifida or pectus excavatum. More frequently, though, this is an elective procedure, to achieve more bulk in the chest area. Sometimes, no matter how much you work out, you cannot develop your pectoral mus-

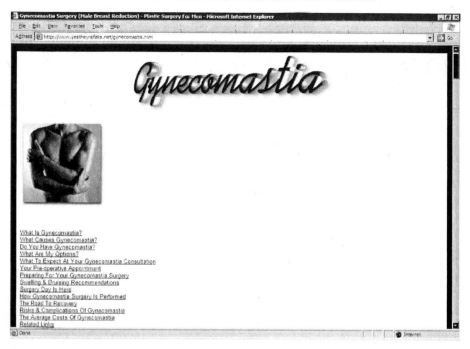

FIGURE 6.3. Yes They're Fake!—Gynecomastia
<http://www.yestheyrefake.net/gynecomastia.html>
Reprinted with permission of Enhancement Media.

cles to reach the appearance that you wish to achieve. This is why many men elect to have pectoral implants. Although this procedure adds size/bulk to the chest, you will still need to exercise to create muscle definition. A search of the Internet for "pectoral augmentation" and "pectoral implant" each found over 29,000 hits. Some of the obvious sites specifically dedicated to pectoral augmentation looked good on initial examination, but were not included here because the source of the information could not be determined.

2004 statistics:

ASAPS: 719   (all male)
ASPS: N/A

BodyImplants.com—Pec Implants (Pectoral Augmentation)
<http://www.bodyimplants.com/pec_implants.html>

This is the site of Dr. Robert Gutstein, a board-certified cosmetic surgeon who specializes in "muscle contouring surgery—cosmetic surgery procedures for both men and women." Pectoral implants/augmentation, one of these procedures, is performed on men. Despite the focus on the doctor's private practice, this site is listed here because it has useful information about pectoral implants/augmentation, including who makes the best candidate, a description of the procedure and recovery time, risks, and questions to ask your doctor. This site has won several Web site design awards.

iEnhance—Male Pectoral Implants
<http://www.ienhance.com/procedure/default.asp>

From the "List of Procedures" select "Plastic Surgery," then under "Breast" select "Male Pectoral Implants." The page covers information such as benefits of the surgery, the surgical consult, questions to ask your doctor, surgical procedure, risks, recovery, and long-term outcome.

InfoPlasticSurgery.com—Pectoral Augmentation
<http://www.infoplasticsurgery.com/breast/pec-implants.html>

This is the private-practice Web site of Dr. Jean Loftus, a female plastic surgeon located in Cincinnati, Ohio, who is the author of *The Smart Woman's Guide to Plastic Surgery*. Dr. Loftus is an advocate for patient education in plastic surgery. The page on pectoral augmentation is the only page on this site aimed at men. It includes information about the surgery, recovery after the surgery, possible complications, costs, and some tips specific to this procedure. Despite the remainder of the site being focused on cosmetic surgery for women, it's worth it for men to check it out, as most of the procedures are similar in men.

Pec Implants.com—Pec Implants (Pectoral Augmentation)
<http://www.pecimplants.com/pecimplants.html>

This site is provided by Dr. Smith, who specializes in cosmetic surgery involving muscle contouring. Information about pectoral implants is given on this page, and another page has information on bicep and tricep implants. This site is included here because it has useful information about the procedure of pectoral augmentation that was not located elsewhere. However, the site is missing any information about Dr. Smith's qualifications—even where the practice is located, so inclusion here is not an endorsement.

Yes They're Fake!—Pectoral Implants
<http://www.yestheyrefake.net/pectoral_implants.html>

The page on pectoral implants (see Figure 6.4) describes the types of implants used and the surgical procedure, recovery, risks, and complications, and price. Preoperative and postoperative instructions are listed, along with photos.

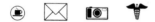

PENIS ENLARGEMENT/IMPLANTS (PHALLOPLASTY)

Who hasn't received an e-mail about penis enlargement? These are an automatic "delete" from my e-mail without even opening them. Advertisements abound on the Internet, on pornography sites, in magazines, and elsewhere about various methods for enlarging the penis. All of these ads are aimed at a man's insecurities about the size of his penis, making an assumption that bigger is better, that penis size is related to sexual performance, and that somehow penis size influences how others view you—or how you view yourself.

Penis enlargement (phalloplasty) can involve enlargement of both the length and width (girth) of the penis. Nonsurgical methods, including drugs and various devices, are often advertised; however, none have been approved for this purpose by the U.S. Food and Drug Administration

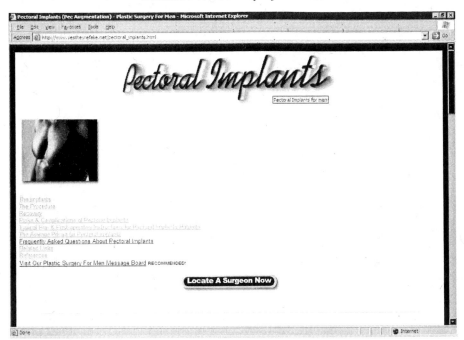

FIGURE 6.4. Yes They're Fake!—Pectoral Implants
<http://www.yestheyrefake.net/pectoral_implants.html>
Reprinted with permission of Enhancement Media.

(FDA). Several surgical techniques are available, including cutting the ligament (increases length), injecting fat (increases width), and grafting blood vessels. None of these techniques are endorsed by any professional medical association.

As noted in several of the Web sites listed in this section, penis enlargement surgery for cosmetic purposes alone is discouraged. However, because there are so many sites about penis enlargement out there on the Internet, it is important to offer a variety of reputable sites to try to offer a balanced view of this procedure. A search for "penis enlargement" via Google resulted in hits—an enormous number of sites; however, quite frankly, most of them were bordering on the pornographic. If you are considering this procedure, please heed the warnings and information contained in the sites listed in this section.

American Society for Aesthetic Plastic Surgery—"Men: Penile Augmentation By Fat Injection—ASAPS Position"
<http://www.surgery.org/press/news-release.php?iid=19>

This ASAPS position statement, issued as a news release, indicates that "enlargement of the penis by fat injection is considered an experimental high-risk procedure." Patients are cautioned to be fully informed of potential risks, to check physician credentials, and to seek a second opinion.

MayoClinic.com—Beware of Penis-Enlargement Scams
<http://www.mayoclinic.com/>

On this site, go to the URL and search for "penis enlargement" to find this article, which discusses both surgical and nonsurgical enlargement of the penis. The article indicates that enlargement procedures are not endorsed by any reputable medical society, and that the American Urological Association, the ASAPS, and the ASPS have policy statements against surgical enhancement of the penis. This is a frank article that warns against the procedure.

New York Phallo
<http://drwhitehead.com>
<http://www.penile-enlargement-surgeon.com>

This Web site gives a detailed description of the surgical enlargement of the penis, which "was popularized in the U.S. in 1991." The page contains graphic anatomical drawings and describes both lengthening and widening, including liposuction and fat injection. This is the page of Dr. E. Douglas Whitehead, president of the American Academy of Phalloplasty Surgeons. This organization was "formed to learn the latest surgical techniques, to network and collaborate, and to disseminate information to the public." The organization itself does not appear to have a Web page of its own, but is mentioned on the Web pages of several private practices, including this one. Dr. Whitehead's credentials (he is Associate Clinical Professor of Urology at Albert Einstein College of Medicine, and holds several other clinical appointments and professional memberships) are prominently listed. This site is obviously intended for prospective patients of this private practice; it has fairly detailed information about the surgical procedure and thus offers information to all men considering this procedure.

Penis-Enlargement.com
<http://www.penis-enlargement.com>

This site indicates that it offers "expert advice for men by the world's leading phalloplasty surgeon." It is the site of Dr. Stephen X. Giunta, a board certified physician who specialized in facial, head and neck plastic surgery and who now offers phalloplasty. His private practice, Aesthetic Plastic Surgery International, in Alexandria, Virginia, is Joint Commission on Accreditation of Healthcare Organizations (JCAHO) approved. He is a member of the American Academy of Phalloplasty Surgeons, which has its own one-page description (this organization does not have its own Web site). This site has detailed information about penis enlargement surgery (widening and lengthening), before-and-after photos, and a comparison of surgery versus other enlargement methods. Although the site is an obvious advertisement for the private practice, it offers a lot of information about the procedure.

UrologyHealth.org
<http://urologyhealth.org/>

This is the patient information site of the American Urological Association. A search on "penile augmentation" locates a basic statement from the AUA that the injection of fat cells and cutting of the suspensory ligament are not yet considered safe procedures.

Yes They're Fake!—Phalloplasty
<http://www.yestheyrefake.net/phalloplasty_penis_enlargement.html>

The page on phalloplasty (penis enlargement) can be located directly via the URL, or, go to the main page <http://www.yestheyrefake.net>, select "Body Procedures" and then "Phalloplasty (Penis Enlargement)." The page describes options for the procedure, along with risks, and recommends a careful choice in surgeons.

Chapter 7

Cosmetic Surgery
of the Face, Head, and Neck

This chapter covers cosmetic surgical procedures of the face, head, and neck. Hair transplantation can be found in Chapter 9. Nonsurgical cosmetic procedures involving primarily the skin, such as laser resurfacing and dermabrasion, can be found in Chapter 8, "Cosmetic Surgery of the Skin." Because there is an overlap with procedures involving the face and skin, cross-references will direct you to appropriate sections in this chapter or to other chapters. Those sites that focus either on the face, head, and neck, or have a special page that groups these procedures together, are listed in the general section. These sites may be listed again along with additional sites under individual procedures.

Statistics from cosmetic surgery associations indicate that over the past five years men are increasingly electing to have cosmetic procedures of the face, head, and neck. Statistics for 2004 show that between 20 and 55 percent of the procedures listed in this chapter were preformed on men. Many of the Web sites are directed toward women because of the larger market, but information about the procedures is relevant to both sexes.

FACE, HEAD, AND NECK—GENERAL

American Academy of Facial Plastic and Reconstructive Surgery
<http://www.aafprs.org>

The AAFPRS Web site says "Trust Your Face to a Facial Plastic Surgeon." In the "Patients" section you'll find information about the society

Internet Guide to Cosmetic Surgery for Men
© 2006 by The Haworth Press, Inc. All rights reserved.
doi:10.1300/5854_08

and an online magazine, but you will want to select "Procedures." From that page you can select the "Virtual Exam Room," which allows you to highlight the part of the face that you want surgery on, and then you can get information on the procedure. "Procedure Types" (see Figure 7.1) links you directly to information on facial surgical procedures that are online adaptations of the academy's brochures. FAQs include some statistics on facial plastic surgery for men, while the glossary defines technical medical terms. This site also has a "Physician Finder."

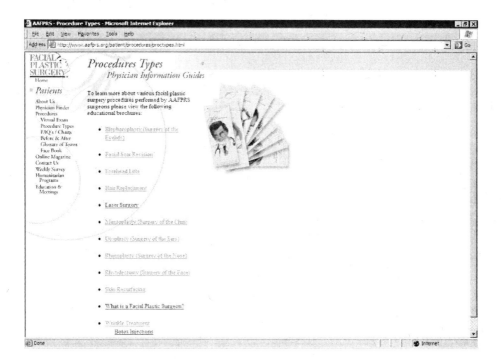

FIGURE 7.1. American Academy of Facial Plastic and Reconstructive Surgery—
    Procedure Types
<http://www.aafprs.org/patient/procedures/proctypes.html>
Reprinted with permission of the American Academy of Facial Plastic and Reconstructive Surgery.

Facial Plastic Surgery Network
<http://www.facialplasticsurgery.net>

"The Facial Plastic Surgery Network is dedicated to helping you obtain solutions to your facial aesthetic concerns." This site is produced by Enhancement Media, a company that has a group of related sites on cosmetic surgery topics. The site is easy to navigate, with links at the top of the home page to "Facial Procedures," "Choosing a Surgeon," "Procedure FAQ," "Anesthesia Information," a photo gallery, chat groups and discussion forums, and more. A key page is "Facial Procedures," which has links to an extensive list of procedures. Some of these are individually listed later in this chapter and also in Chapter 8 "Cosmetic Surgery of the Skin." Information is similar to the site **Yes They're Fake!** which is produced by the same company, just without the candid commentary.

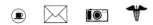

iEnhance—Facial Plastic Surgery
<http://www.ienhance.com/speciality/facial.asp>

Go directly to the page (*sic*—speciality in URL), or begin at the general <http://www.ienhance.com> and select "Facial Plastic Surgery." This page has links to featured articles, archived articles, a photo gallery, a doctor locator, and specific surgical procedures. Select "Procedures" from this page, and then "Facial Plastic Surgery" to link to information on twenty-five to thirty facial plastic surgery procedures, from eyelid surgery to lip augmentation (see Figure 7.2). Also included here are skin procedures (see Chapter 8, "Cosmetic Surgery of the Skin") and hair transplantation (see Chapter 9, "Hair Transplantation for Men").

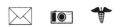

Yes They're Fake!—Facial Enhancement
<http://www.yestheyrefake.net/facial_plastic_surgery.html>

Many of the specific procedures from this "Facial Enhancement" page are listed later in this chapter (or in Chapter 8, "Cosmetic Surgery of the Skin") under the specific procedure, but it was not possible to list all.

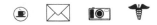

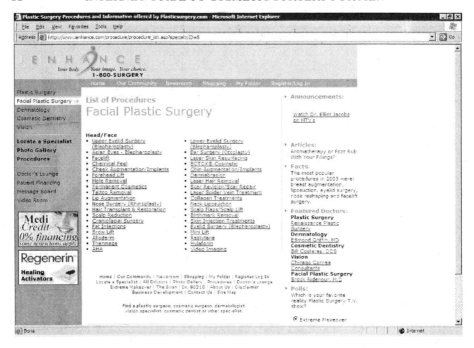

FIGURE 7.2. iEnhance—Facial Plastic Surgery
<http://www.ienhance.com/procedure/procedure_list.asp?specialtyID=5>
Reprinted with permission of iEnhance.com.

BLEPHAROPLASTY

See EYELID SURGERY (BLEPHAROPLASTY) (in this chapter).

BOTULINUM TOXIN (BOTOX) INJECTIONS

See Chapter 8, "Cosmetic Surgery of the Skin."

BROW LIFT

See FOREHEAD LIFT (BROW LIFT) (in this chapter).

BUCCAL FAT PAD REMOVAL

This procedure removes the fat pads in the lower cheeks to give a more defined look to the cheeks.

Facial Plastic Surgery Network—Buccal Fat Pad Extraction <http://www.facialplasticsurgery.net/buccal_fat.htm>

This page (see Figure 7.3) describes the surgical procedure, expectations, recovery, risks and complications, and more.

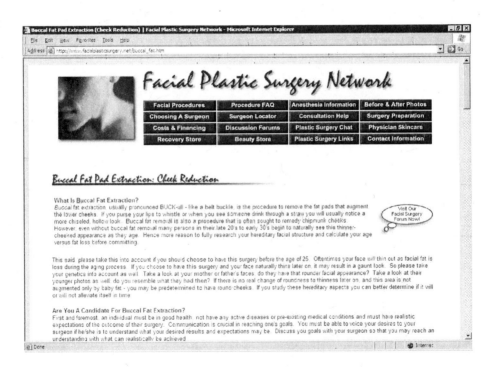

FIGURE 7.3. Facial Plastic Surgery Network—Buccal Fat Pad Extraction <http://www.facialplasticsurgery.net/buccal_fat.htm>
Reprinted with permission of Enhancement Media.

Yes They're Fake!—Buccal Fat Pad Removal
<http://www.yestheyrefake.net/buccal_fat.htm>

The page on buccal fat pad removal describes the procedure (removing fat pads in the cheeks—"chipmunk cheeks"), whether you are a candidate for this surgery, the recovery, risks and complications, and more.

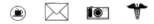

CHEEK IMPLANTS (AUGMENTATION)

See also FACIAL IMPLANTS (in this chapter).

Cheek implants are used to augment or increase the size of the cheek bones, giving a more defined look to the cheeks.

2004 statistics:

ASAPS:	10,883	(2,006 in men)
ASPS:	9,318	(3,914 in men)

All About Cheek Augmentation
<http://www.cheekaugmentation.com>

This site is easy to navigate with links to "About Cheek Augmentation" (includes whether you are a candidate for the surgery, risks, complications, and photo gallery), "Your Options & More" (includes anesthesia and incision placement), "The Surgery," "Road to Recovery" (includes what to expect and complications), and more. Included in "Surgeon Information" are tips on how to choose a good surgeon and how to research the surgeon's credentials.

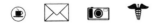

iEnhance—Cheek Augmentation/Implants
<http://www.ienhance.com/procedure/default.asp>

From the "List of Procedures," select either "Plastic Surgery" or "Facial Plastic Surgery," then under "Head/Face" select "Cheek Augmentation/ Implants." The page includes basic information such as patient selection, surgical procedure, risks, postsurgical recovery, and questions to ask your doctor.

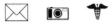

Yes They're Fake!—Cheek Augmentation
<http://www.yestheyrefake.net/cheek_augmentation.htm>

The page on cheek augmentation helps you decide if you are a candidate for chin surgery, lists surgical options and postsurgical recovery, and risks, complications, and contraindications. You are referred to **All About Cheek Augmentation <http://www.cheekaugmentation.com>** for more information.

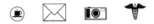

CHEEK REDUCTION

See BUCCAL FAT PAD REMOVAL (in this chapter).

CHEMICAL PEELS

See Chapter 8, "Cosmetic Surgery of the Skin."

CHIN AUGMENTATION (MENTOPLASTY)

See also FACIAL IMPLANTS (in this chapter).

Chin augmentation involves placing an implant over the bone and under the skin. This procedure is done for individuals who have a "weak" chin. By increasing the size of the chin, the face is given better balance and the profile is improved. Chin augmentation is often done in conjunction with nose surgery or facial liposuction.

2004 statistics:

ASAPS: 32,039 (7,958 in men)
ASPS: 15,822 (8,860 in men)

All About Chin Augmentation
<http://www.chinaugmentation.com>

This site is easy to navigate with links for "About Chin Augmentation" (includes whether you are a candidate for the surgery, risks, complications, and photo gallery), "Your Options & More" (includes anesthesia and incision placement), "The Surgery," "Road to Recovery" (includes what to expect and complications), and more. Included in "Surgeon Information" are tips on how to choose a good surgeon and how to research the surgeon's credentials.

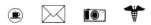

American Academy of Facial Plastic and Reconstructive Surgery—
   Understanding Mentoplasty Surgery
<http://www.aafprs.org/patient/procedures/mentoplasty.html>

The AAFPRS patient information page (see Figure 7.4) includes a description of the procedure, deciding on chin surgery, postsurgery information, and before/after illustrations.

American Society of Plastic Surgeons—Chin Surgery
<http://www.plasticsurgery.org/public_education/procedures/
   Mentoplasty.cfm>

The ASPS information page has only brief information about chin surgery. Check also the ASPS page on Facial Implants (Chin, Cheeks & Jaw Surgery), <http://www.plasticsurgery.org/public_education/procedures/FacialImplants.cfm>.

iEnhance—Chin Augmentation/Implants
<http://www.ienhance.com/procedure/default.asp>

From the "List of Procedures" select either "Plastic Surgery" or "Facial Plastic Surgery," then under "Head/Face" select "Chin Augmentation/

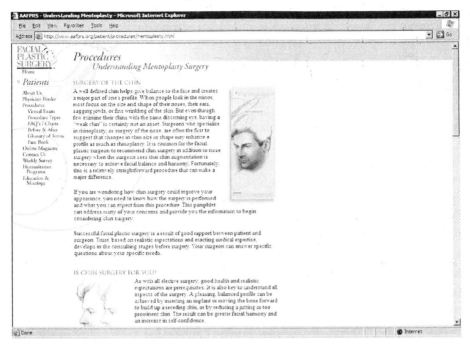

FIGURE 7.4. American Academy of Facial Plastic and Reconstructive Surgery—
  Understanding Mentoplasty Surgery
<http://www.aafprs.org/patient/procedures/mentoplasty.html>
Reprinted with permission of American Academy of Facial Plastic and Reconstructive
  Surgery.

Implants." The page includes basic information such as patient selection,
surgical procedure, risks, postsurgical recovery, and questions to ask your
doctor.

Yes They're Fake!—Chin Augmentation
<http://www.yestheyrefake.net/chin_augmentation.htm>

The page on chin augmentation helps you decide if you are a candidate
for chin surgery, lists surgical options and postsurgical recovery, and risks,

complications, and contraindications. You are referred to **All About Chin Augmentation <http://www.chinaugmentation.com>** for more information.

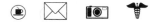

DERMABRASION

See Chapter 8, "Cosmetic Surgery of the Skin."

EAR SURGERY (OTOPLASTY)

Otoplasty is the surgical procedure used to correct ears that protrude or stick out from the side of the head, or to reduce the size of the ears. Commonly called "pinning back" the ears, otoplasty improves one's appearance without affecting the hearing. This is one of the most popular cosmetic procedures for men.

2004 statistics:

ASAPS: 26,366   (10,628 in men)
ASPS: 25,915   (11,403 in men)

American Academy of Facial Plastic and Reconstructive Surgery— Understanding Otoplasty Surgery
<http://www.aafprs.org/patient/procedures/otoplasty.html>

The AAFPRS patient information page (see Figure 7.5) includes a description of the procedure, deciding on ear surgery, and postsurgery information, and also includes illustrations.

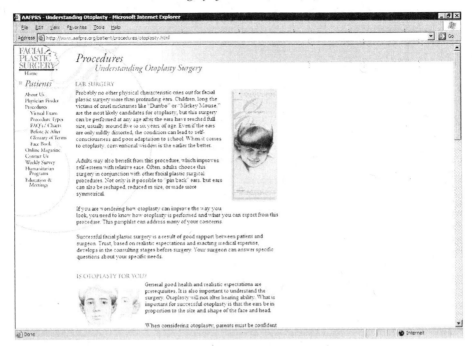

FIGURE 7.5. American Academy of Facial Plastic and Reconstructive Surgery—
Understanding Otoplasty Surgery
<http://aafprs.org/patient/procedures.otoplasty.html>
Reprinted with permission of American Academy of Facial Plastic and Reconstructive
Surgery.

American Academy of Otolaryngology—Head and Neck Surgery—
Ear Plastic Surgery
<http://www.entnet.org/healthinfo/ears/plastic_surgery.cfm>

The AAO-HNS page discusses pinning back the ears, correcting ear deformities, and torn earlobes.

American Society of Plastic Surgeons—Otoplasty (Ear Surgery)
<http://www.plasticsurgery.org/public_education/procedures/
  otoplasty.cfm>

The ASPS public information page on ear surgery includes a description of the surgery, anesthesia, risks, postsurgical recovery, and before/after illustrations.

Bermant Plastic and Cosmetic Surgery—Otoplasty Cosmetic
  Sculpture of the Ears
<http://www.plasticsurgery4u.com/procedure_folder/ears/index.html>

This site is provided by Dr. Michael Bermant, a board-certified physician in plastic surgery, who practices near Richmond, Virginia. The site contains a wealth of information. A strength of the otoplasty page is the links to photos of male otoplasty patients. The site subscribes to the HONcode principles.

Facial Plastic Surgery Network—Otoplasty (Ear Pinning,
  Reshaping)
<http://www.facialplasticsurgery.net/otoplasty.htm>

The otoplasty page contains a description of the procedure, helps you decide whether you are a candidate for surgery, and discusses expectations, recovery, risks and complications, etc.

iEnhance—Ear Surgery (Otoplasty)
<http://www.ienhance.com/procedure/default.asp>

From the "List of Procedures" select either "Plastic Surgery" or "Facial Plastic Surgery," then under "Head/Face" select "Ear Surgery (Otoplasty)."

This page includes basic information such as patient selection, surgical procedure, risks, postsurgical recovery, and questions to ask your doctor.

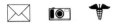

Yes They're Fake!—Otoplasty
<http://www.yestheyrefake.net/otoplasty.htm>

The page on otoplasty helps you decide if you are a candidate for otoplasty (which is described here as ear pinning), describes preparing for surgery, the surgical procedure, postsurgical recovery, and lists risks and complications.

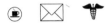

EYELID SURGERY (BLEPHAROPLASTY)

Blepharoplasty is cosmetic surgery of the eyelids. It removes the excess fat from the upper and lower eyelids. The procedure corrects droopy eyelids and can remove the "bags" from under your eyes. Blepharoplasty is often done with other cosmetic surgery of the face, such as a facelift or skin resurfacing.

2004 statistics:

ASAPS: 290,343 (41,050 in men)
ASPS: 233,334 (32,667 in men)

American Academy of Facial Plastic and Reconstructive Surgery—
    Understanding Blepharoplasty
<http://www.aafprs.org/patient/procedures/blepharoplasty.html>

The AAFPRS site discusses making the decision to have blepharoplasty, the surgery, and what to expect postsurgery. Before/after illustrations are included.

American Society for Aesthetic Plastic Surgery—Eyelid Surgery
<http://www.surgery.org/public/procedures-eyelid.php>

This ASAPS public page on eyelid surgery leads to additional pages containing information about the surgical procedure, risks, before and after surgery, and more. This is one of the better sites available about eyelid surgery.

 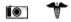

American Society for Dermatologic Surgery—Aging Eyelids
<http://www.asds.net/Patients/FactSheets/patients-Fact_Sheet-
aging_eyelids.html>

This ASDS fact sheet about aging eyelids describes blepharoplasty, including information about the procedure, postoperative effects, and complications.

American Society of Plastic Surgeons—Blepharoplasty
(Eyelids)
<http://www.plasticsurgery.org/public_education/procedures/
Blepharoplasty.cfm>

The ASPS public information page on eyelid surgery includes a description of the surgery, anesthesia, risks, postsurgical recovery, and before/after illustrations. This page is available in Spanish (choose Spanish from Procedures page or go directly to <http://www.plasticsurgery.org/public_education/procedures/Blefaroplastia.cfm>).

Bermant Plastic and Cosmetic Surgery—Blepharoplasty Eyelid Cosmetic Surgery
<http://www.plasticsurgery4u.com/procedure_folder/blepharoplasty/index.html>

This site by Dr. Michael Bermant contains a wealth of information. Go directly to the URL or scroll on the main page until you get to "Eyelid Sculpture" and then link to information about blepharoplasty. The site subscribes to the HONcode principles.

Facial Plastic Surgery Network—Blepharoplasty: Eyelid Tuck Surgery
<http://www.facialplasticsurgery.net/blepharoplasty.htm>

This page describes the procedure for blepharoplasty, including expectations, recovery, risks and complications, and more.

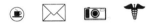

iEnhance—Eyelid Surgery (Blepharoplasty)
<http://www.ienhance.com/procedure/default.asp>

From the "List of Procedures" select either "Plastic Surgery" or "Facial Plastic Surgery," then, under "Head/Face" are four separate pages: "Upper Eyelid Surgery (Blepharoplasty)," "Lower Eyelid Surgery (Blepharoplasty)," "Eyelid Surgery (Blepharoplasty)," and "Asian Eyes-Blepharoplasty." The general blepharoplasty page has little information, but the other three include basic information such as patient selection, surgical procedure, risks, postsurgical recovery, and questions to ask your doctor.

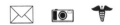

Yes They're Fake!—Blepharoplasty
<http://www.yestheyrefake.net/blepharoplasty.htm>

The page on blepharoplasty helps you decide if you are a candidate for blepharoplasty (eyelid surgery or eyelid lift), describes preparing for surgery, the surgical procedure, and postsurgical recovery, and lists risks and complications.

FACELIFT (RHYTIDECTOMY)

Rhytidectomy is the technical name for a facelift. Facelifts are performed to reduce the effects of aging by removing wrinkles that form in the skin, along with the removal of excess fat and tightening of the muscles. Facelifts are often performed along with eyelid surgery, a forehead lift, and other facial cosmetic procedures.

2004 statistics:

ASAPS: 157,061 (11,821 in men)
ASPS: 114,279 (10,285 in men)

American Academy of Facial Plastic and Reconstructive Surgery— Understanding Rhytidectomy
<http://www.aafprs.org/patient/procedures/rhytidectomy.html>

The AAFPRS patient information includes a description of the procedure, deciding on a facelift, and postsurgery information, and also includes before/after illustrations.

American Society for Aesthetic Plastic Surgery—Facelift
<http://www.surgery.org/public/procedures-facelift.php>

The ASAPS public page on facelift surgery leads to additional pages containing information about the surgical procedure, risks, before and after surgery, and more. This is one of the better sites available about facelift surgery.

 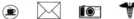

American Society of Plastic Surgeons—Rhytidectomy (Facelift) <http://www.plasticsurgery.org/public_education/procedures/ rhytidectomy.cfm>

This ASPS public information page on facelift (see Figure 7.6) includes a description of the surgery, anesthesia, risks, postsurgical recovery, and before/after illustrations. This page is available in Spanish (choose Spanish from Procedures page or go directly to <http://www.plasticsurgery. org/public_education/procedures/Ritidectomia.cfm>).

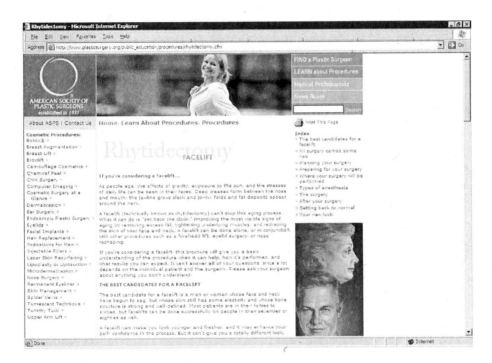

FIGURE 7.6. American Society of Plastic Surgeons—Rhytidectomy (Facelift) <http://www.plasticsurgery.org/public_education/procedures/rhytidectomy.cfm> ©2004 American Society of Plastic Surgeons. All rights reserved. Learn more at <www.plasticsurgery.org>.

Bermant Plastic and Cosmetic Surgery—Facelift Surgery
<http://www.plasticsurgery4u.com>

This is the site of Dr. Michael Bermant, a board certified physician in plastic surgery, who practices near Richmond, Virginia. Scroll until you get to "Facelift Surgery," located in the "Sculpture of the Face" section. Links go to pages on facelift, neck lift, and brow lift. The "Site Search" feature is also useful. The site subscribes to the HONcode principles.

Facelift FYI
<http://www.faceliftfyi.com>

A special section of the CosmeticSurgeryFYI Web site, this site gives extensive information about facelifts, including the surgical procedure, who is a candidate for surgery, and risks. The site contains links to before/after photos. The commercial aspect is evident with a link to the surgeon locator on each page, plus financing information.

Facial Plastic Surgery Network—Face Lift
<http://www.facialplasticsurgery.net/face_lift.htm>

This page includes information about the types of facelifts, a procedure description, expectations, recovery, risks and complications, and more.

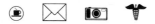

iEnhance—FaceLift
<http://www.ienhance.com/procedure/default.asp>

From the "List of Procedures" select either "Plastic Surgery" or "Facial Plastic Surgery," then under "Head/Face" select "FaceLift." The page includes basic information such as patient selection, surgical procedure, risks, postsurgical recovery, and questions to ask your doctor, and also discusses facelifts in relation to other procedures such as eyelid surgery and skin resurfacing.

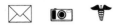

MayoClinic.com—Saving Face: The Nips and Tucks of Face-Lifts <http://www.mayoclinic.com/>

Go to the general Mayo site and do a site search for "face lift" to locate the page on "Saving Face." This page cautions prospective patients to have a realistic expectation of results, describes the procedure and postsurgical effects, along with risks.

Yes They're Fake!—Face Lift <http://www.yestheyrefake.net/face_lift.htm>

The page on Face Lift describes the underlying facial structure, whether you are a candidate for a facelift, the types of facelifts, preparing for surgery and the recovery, risks and complications, questions to ask, and more. Also check out the link to "Feather Lift (APTOS Threads)" from the "Facial Procedures" page, or go directly to <http://www.yestheyrefake.net/feather_lift.htm>.

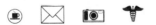

FACIAL IMPLANTS

Facial implants alter and enhance the shape of your face and are most commonly performed on the cheekbones and chin (*see also* CHEEK IMPLANTS (AUGMENTATION), CHIN AUGMENTATION, and JAW AUGMENTATION in this chapter). The implants may be done in conjunction with other cosmetic procedures of the face, such as facelifts or rhinoplasty (surgery of the nose).

2004 statistics:

ASAPS: 10,883 cheek implants   (2,006 in men)
ASPS: 9,318 cheek implants   (3,914 in men)

American Society for Aesthetic Plastic Surgery—Facial Implants
<http://www.surgery.org/public/procedures-faceimplants.php>

This ASAPS public page on facial implants (see Figure 7.7) describes the surgical technique, benefits, and risks of facial implants.

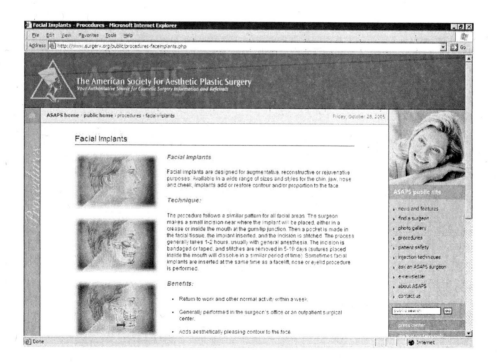

FIGURE 7.7. American Society for Aesthetic Plastic Surgery—Facial Implants <http://www.surgery.org/public/procedures-faceimplants.php> Reprinted with permission of American Society of Aesthetic Plastic Surgery.

American Society of Plastic Surgeons—Facial Implants (Chin, Cheeks and Jaw Surgery)
<http://www.plasticsurgery.org/public_education/procedures/ facialimplants.cfm>

The ASPS public information page on facial implants includes a description of the surgery, anesthesia, risks, postsurgical recovery, and before/ after illustrations. Chin, cheek, and lower jaw surgery procedures are discussed.

Yes They're Fake!—Facial Implants
<http://www.yestheyrefake.net/facial_implants.htm>

The page on facial implants primarily discusses five implant products: Advanta Facial Implant, Gore-Tex Facial Implant, Gore-Tex Strands and Multi-Strands, SoftForm, and UltraSoft.

FACIAL LIPOSUCTION

Facial liposuction is the removal of fat from the face and under the chin. The procedure is done to give a more defined look to the face and can be performed in conjunction with other procedures such as a chin implant.

Facial Plastic Surgery Network—Facial & Neck Liposuction
<http://www.facialplasticsurgery.net/facial_liposuction.htm>

This page (see Figure 7.8) describes the surgical procedure, whether you are a candidate for surgery, expectations from the surgery, recovery, risks and complications, and more.

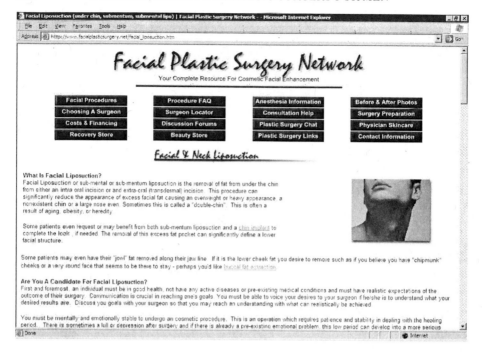

FIGURE 7.8. Facial Plastic Surgery Network—Facial and Submental Liposuction
<http://www.facialplasticsurgery.net/facial_liposuction.htm>
Reprinted with permission of Enhancement Media.

Yes They're Fake!—Facial Liposuction
<http://www.yestheyrefake.net/facial_liposuction.htm>

The page on facial liposuction helps you decide if you are a candidate for facial liposuction, describes the preoperative preparation, the surgery, postsurgical recovery, and lists risks and complications.

FAT INJECTIONS

See FAT INJECTIONS in Chapter 8, "Cosmetic Surgery of the Skin."

FOREHEAD LIFT (BROW LIFT)

A forehead (brow) lift is done to reduce the signs of aging in this area of the face. In the procedure, wrinkles are reduced/eliminated by removing excess skin and, if necessary, part of the underlying muscles. This procedure is frequently done with a facelift and/or eye surgery.

2004 statistics:

ASAPS: 95,212   (8,030 in men)
ASPS: 54,993   (7,699 in men)

American Academy of Facial Plastic and Reconstructive Surgery— Understanding Forehead & Brow Lift Surgery
<http://www.aafprs.org/patient/procedures/forehead_lifts.html>

The AAFPRS patient information includes a description of the procedure, deciding on chin surgery, and postsurgery information; it also includes before/after illustrations.

American Society for Aesthetic Plastic Surgery—Forehead Lift
<http://www.surgery.org/public/procedures-forehead.php>

This is the ASAPS public page on forehead lift; it leads to additional pages containing information about the surgical procedure, risks, before and after surgery, and more. This is one of the better sites available about forehead lifts.

American Society of Plastic Surgeons—Browlift (Forehead Lift)
<http://www.plasticsurgery.org/public_education/procedures/ Browlift.cfm>

This ASPS public information page on surgery of the forehead (see Figure 7.9) includes a description of the surgery, anesthesia, risks, postsurgical recovery, and before/after illustrations.

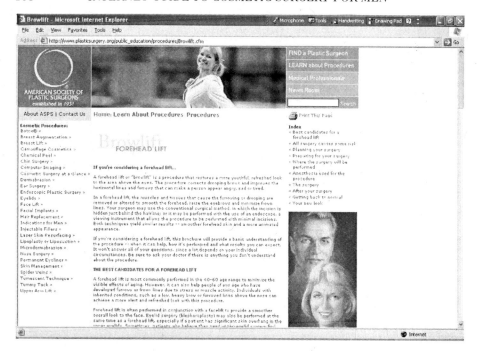

FIGURE 7.9. American Society of Plastic Surgeons—Browlift (Forehead Lift) <http://www.plasticsurgery.org/public_education/procedures/Browlift.cfm> ©2004 American Society of Plastic Surgeons. All rights reserved. Learn more at <www.plasticsurgery.org>.

Bermant Plastic and Cosmetic Surgery—Brow Lift (Forehead Lift) <http://www.plasticsurgery4u.com/procedure_folder/brow_lift.html>

This site of Dr. Michael Bermant contains a wealth of information. Go directly to the URL or scroll until you get to the single line—"Brow Lift the Surgery," and then link to the page on brow lifts. The site subscribes to the HONcode principles.

Facial Plastic Surgery Network—Forehead & Brow Lift Surgery
<http://www.facialplasticsurgery.net/brow_forehead_lift.htm>

This page describes the surgical procedure and what to expect following the surgery, including recovery time, risks and complications, and more.

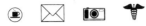

iEnhance—Forehead Lift
<http://www.ienhance.com/procedure/default.asp>

From the "List of Procedures" select either "Plastic Surgery" or "Facial Plastic Surgery," then under "Head/Face" select "Forehead Lift." The page includes basic information such as patient selection, surgical procedure (conventional and endoscopic forehead lift), risks, postsurgical recovery, questions to ask your doctor, and related procedures.

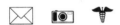

Yes They're Fake!—Brow or Forehead Lift
<http://www.yestheyrefake.net/brow_forehead-lift.htm>

The page on brow/forehead lift helps you decide if you are a candidate for a brow lift, describes the preoperative preparation, the surgery, and postsurgical recovery, and lists risks and complications.

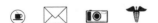

JAW AUGMENTATION

See also FACIAL IMPLANTS (in this chapter).

Jaw augmentation is the cosmetic procedure that increases the size of the jaw (mandible), using a synthetic product. It can be done in conjunction with a chin implant, and also with nose surgery, to give a more balanced look to the face.

All About Jaw Augmentation
<http://www.jawaugmentation.com>

This site is easy to navigate with links for "About Jaw Augmentation" (includes whether you are a candidate for the surgery, risks, complications, and photo gallery), "Your Options & More" (includes anesthesia and incision placement), "The Surgery," "Road to Recovery" (includes what to expect and complications), and more. Included in "Surgeon Information" are tips on how to choose a good surgeon and how to research the surgeon's credentials.

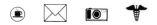

Facial Plastic Surgery Network—Jaw Augmentation
& Jaw Implants
<http://www.facialplasticsurgery.net/jaw_augmentation.htm>

This page on jaw augmentation (see Figure 7.10) helps you decide if you are a candidate for chin surgery, lists surgical options and postsurgical recovery, and lists risks, complications, and contraindications. You are referred to **All About Jaw Augmentation <http://www.jawaugmentation. com>** for more information.

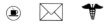

Yes They're Fake!—Jaw Augmentation
<http://www.yestheyrefake.net/jaw_augmentation.htm>

The page on jaw augmentation helps you decide if you are a candidate for jaw surgery, lists surgical options and postsurgical recovery, and lists risks, complications, and contraindications. You are referred to a related site, **All About Jaw Augmentation <http://www.jawaugmentation.com>** for more information.

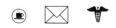

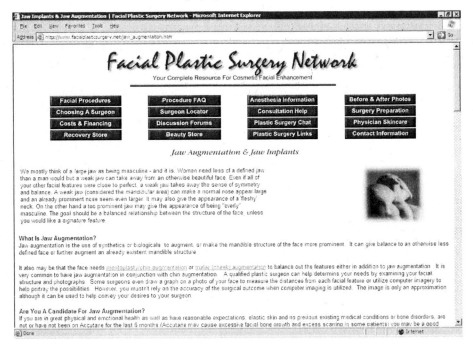

FIGURE 7.10. Facial Plastic Surgery Network—Jaw Augmentation and Jaw Implants
<http://www.facialplasticsurgery.net/jaw_augmentation.htm>
Reprinted with permission of Enhancement Media.

LASER SKIN RESURFACING

See DERMABRASION, LASER SKIN RESURFACING, and CHEMICAL PEELS in Chapter 8, "Cosmetic Surgery of the Skin."

LIP AUGMENTATION

See also INJECTABLE FILLERS in Chapter 8, "Cosmetic Surgery of the Skin."

Lip augmentation increases the size of your lips. This procedure involves inserting a synthetic filler or injecting natural materials, and is used to augment the size of the lips or to battle the signs of aging. Upper, lower, or both lips can be augmented. Lip augmentation is a relatively rare procedure in men.

2004 statistics:

ASAPS: 30,804 (other than injectable materials)   (499 in men)
ASPS: 26,730 (other than injectable material)   (802 in men)

All About Lip Augmentation
<http://www.lipaugmentation.com>

This easy-to-navigate site has links to "Understanding Your Lips" (includes anatomy), "About Lip Augmentation" (includes risks, complications, and photo gallery), "Procedure Information," and more. Included in "Surgeon Information" are tips on how to choose a good surgeon and how to research the surgeon's credentials.

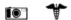

American Society for Aesthetic Plastic Surgery—Lip Augmentation
<http://www.surgery.org/public/procedures-lipaug.php>

The ASAPS public page on lip augmentation contains general information about the procedure, a description of the technique, options to consider, benefits, and other considerations.

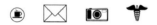

iEnhance—Lip Augmentation
<http://www.ienhance.com/procedure/default.asp>

From the "List of Procedures" select either "Plastic Surgery" or "Facial Plastic Surgery," then under "Head/Face" select "Lip Augmentation." The page includes basic information such as patient selection, surgical procedure, risks, postsurgical recovery, and questions to ask your doctor.

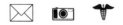

Yes They're Fake!—Lip Augmentation
<http://www.yestheyrefake.net/lip_augmentation.html>

The page on lip augmentation will help you to determine if you are a candidate for lip surgery, lists surgical options, postsurgical recovery, and risks, complications, and contraindications.

LIP REDUCTION

Lip reduction can be done for patients who feel that their lips are too large and wish to reduce their size. The procedure involves removing tissue from the lips (either the upper or lower lip, or both lips).

Facial Plastic Surgery Network—Lip Reduction
<http://www.facialplasticsurgery.net/lip_reduction.htm>

The lip reduction page includes information about the surgical procedure, how to determine whether you are a candidate for surgery, expectations, recovery, risks, and complications, etc.

Yes They're Fake!—Lip Reduction
<http://www.yestheyrefake.net/lip_reduction.htm>

The page on lip reduction helps you decide if you are a candidate for lip surgery, describes the surgery and postsurgical recovery, and lists risks and complications.

MENTOPLASTY

See CHIN AUGMENTATION (MENTOPLASTY) (in this chapter). *See also* FACIAL IMPLANTS (in this chapter).

MICRODERMABRASION

See MICRODERMABRASION in Chapter 8, "Cosmetic Surgery of the Skin."

NECK LIFT/NECK LIPOSUCTION

A neck lift is surgery that reduces/removes the sagging skin of the neck or removes excess fat in the neck area, giving the jaw a more defined look and eliminating wrinkles. A neck lift is often performed in conjunction with a facelift or other facial procedures.

Facial Plastic Surgery Network—Neck Lift (Platysmaplasty)
<http://www.facialplasticsurgery.net/neck_lift.htm>

The page on neck lifts helps you decide whether you are a candidate for surgery, and then describes the surgical procedure, expectations, recovery, risks, and complications, etc.

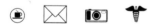

iEnhance—Neck Liposuction
<http://www.ienhance.com/procedure/default.asp>

From the "List of Procedures" select either "Plastic Surgery" or "Facial Plastic Surgery," then under "Head/Face" select "Neck Liposuction." The page includes basic information such as whether you are a candidate for surgery, surgical procedure, risks, postsurgical recovery, and questions to ask your doctor.

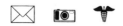

Yes They're Fake!—Neck Lift
<http://www.yestheyrefake.net/neck_lift.htm>

The page on neck lift (platysmaplasty) describes what a neck lift is, whether you are a candidate for a neck lift, how the surgery is performed, the recovery, risks and complications, and more.

NOSE SURGERY (RHINOPLASTY)

Rhinoplasty, or surgery of the nose ("nose job"), is performed for both cosmetic purposes, i.e., to improve your appearance, or for functional reasons, i.e., to improve breathing. Reshaping of the nose—changing the size and shape—has a major impact on one's appearance, and thus it is one of the most common cosmetic procedures.

2004 statistics:

ASAPS: 166,187   (38,989 in men)
ASPS: 305,475   (109,971 in men)

American Academy of Facial Plastic and Reconstructive Surgery—
Understanding Rhinoplasty Surgery
<http://www.aafprs.org/patient/procedures/rhinoplasty.html>

The AAFPRS patient information includes a description of the procedure, deciding on nose surgery, postsurgery information, and before/after illustrations.

American Academy of Otolaryngology—Head and Neck Surgery—Surgery of the Nose
<http://www.entnet.org/healthinfo/nose/surgery_nose.cfm>

The AAO-HNS site discusses surgery of the nose both for cosmetic and functional reasons (e.g., nasal obstruction). Before/after illustrations are available.

American Society for Aesthetic Plastic Surgery—Nose Reshaping
<http://www.surgery.org/public/procedures-nosereshape.php>

This ASAPS public page on nose reshaping leads to additional pages containing information about the surgical procedure, risks, before and after surgery, and more. This is one of the better sites available about rhinoplasty.

American Society of Plastic Surgeons—Rhinoplasty (Surgery of the Nose)
<http://www.plasticsurgery.org/public_education/procedures/Rhinoplasty.cfm>

The ASPS public information page on surgery of the nose (see Figure 7.11) includes a description of the surgery, anesthesia, risks, postsurgical recovery, and before/after illustrations. This page is available in Spanish (choose Spanish from the Procedures page or go directly to <http://www.plasticsurgery.org/public_education/procedures/Rinoplastia.cfm>).

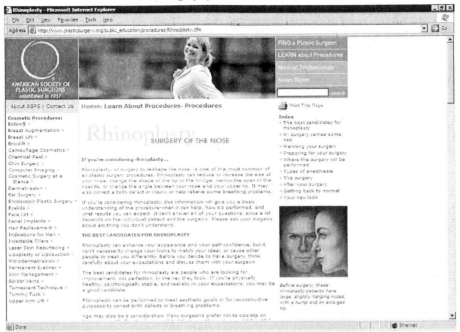

FIGURE 7.11. American Society of Plastic Surgeons—Rhinoplasty (Surgery of the Nose) <http://www.plasticsurgery.org/public_education/procedures/Rhinoplasty.cfm> ©2004 American Society of Plastic Surgeons. All rights reserved. Learn more at <www.plasticsurgery.org>.

Bermant Plastic and Cosmetic Surgery—Male Rhinoplasty <http://www.plasticsurgery4u.com/procedure_folder/nose/male_ rhinoplasty.html>

This site by Dr. Michael Bermant is a bit disorganized, but it contains a wealth of information. Go directly to the URL, or scroll down the home page until you get to "Nasal Sculpture" and then link to information about rhinoplasty, from the procedure itself to ethnic issues. From the rhinoplasty/nasal sculpture page, select "Male Rhinoplasty Patients" to get to <http://www.plasticsurgry4u.com/procedure_folder/nose/male_rhinoplasty. html>, which includes before and after photos. The site subscribes to the HONcode principles.

iEnhance—Nose Surgery (Rhinoplasty)
<http://www.ienhance.com/procedure/default.asp>

From the "List of Procedures" select either "Plastic Surgery" or "Facial Plastic Surgery," then under "Head/Face" select "Nose Surgery (Rhinoplasty)." The page includes basic information such as patient selection, surgical procedure, risks, postsurgical recovery, and questions to ask your doctor.

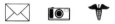

Rhinoplasty 4 You
<http://www.rhinoplasty4you.com>

This site is easy to navigate with links for "Understanding the Nose," "Researching the Procedure" (includes a glossary, surgical procedure details, risks, and complications), "Road to Recovery," a photo gallery (linked under "Miscellaneous Information"), and more.

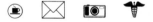

Rhinoplasty FYI
<http://www.rhinoplastyfyi.com>

This is a special section of the CosmeticSurgeryFYI site. It gives extensive information about the rhinoplasty surgical procedure and patient expectations, who is a candidate for surgery, and risks, and contains links to before/after photos. There is a link to the surgeon locator on each page, plus financing information.

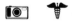

Yes They're Fake!—Rhinoplasty
<http://www.yestheyrefake.net/rhinoplasty.html>

The page on rhinoplasty (nose surgery) discusses whether you are a candidate for rhinoplasty, risks and complications, and depression after rhinoplasty; also included are FAQs about rhinoplasty, a before-and-after photo gallery, and a rhinoplasty message board. Check out the links to "Revision Rhinoplasty" <http://www.yestheyrefake.net/revision_rhinoplasty.htm> and "Septoplasty" <http://www.yestheyrefake.com.septoplasty.htm>. A link refers you to **Rhinoplasty 4 You <http://www.rhinoplasty.com>.**

OTOPLASTY

See EAR SURGERY (OTOPLASTY) (in this chapter).

RHINOPLASTY

See NOSE SURGERY (RHINOPLASTY) (in this chapter).

RHYTIDECTOMY

See FACELIFT (RHYTIDECTOMY) (in this chapter).

Chapter 8

Cosmetic Surgery of the Skin

This chapter reviews information about cosmetic procedures of the skin, covering all parts of the body, including the face. The majority of cosmetic surgery procedures for the skin are designed to combat the aging process, e.g., wrinkles, sagging skin, rough/irregular patches of skin. However, some procedures such as tattoo removal or scar revision are cosmetic in nature, but are not related to aging.

Procedures in this chapter include nonsurgical treatments, laser treatments, resurfacing, and injections. Because so many of these procedures have multiple uses, and many of the conditions have options for treatment, it was difficult to organize this chapter. You are encouraged to browse this entire chapter rather than focus on a specific procedure, as many sites offer different approaches to a topic. Cross-references will direct you to appropriate sections in this or other chapters.

Surgical procedures intended to reshape the face, head, and neck are covered in Chapter 7, "Cosmetic Surgery of the Face, Head, and Neck." Hair replacement is covered in Chapter 9, "Hair Transplantation for Men." If you are unable to locate a procedure, please check the index.

SKIN—GENERAL

AgingSkinNet
<http://www.skincarephysicians.com/agingskinnet/index.html>

AgingSkinNet is "an educational program brought to you by the American Academy of Dermatology." Within this site is a section, "Cosmetic Procedures," which provides brief information about a variety of procedures,

Internet Guide to Cosmetic Surgery for Men
© 2006 by The Haworth Press, Inc. All rights reserved.
doi:10.1300/5854_09

both surgical and nonsurgical, that can be used to treat aging skin. Other pages include information on spider/varicose veins, hair loss, and choosing a dermatologist.

American Academy of Dermatology—Public Resources Center— Pamphlets
<http://www.aad.org/public/Publications/PamphletsIntro.htm>

For patient information from the American Academy of Dermatology, it's best to go directly to the URL. However, if you choose to begin at the home page, <http://www.aad.org> (see Figure 8.1), select "Public Resource Center" and then, on the lower left-hand side of the page, "Publications," followed by "Pamphlets." Pamphlets range from cosmetic surgery

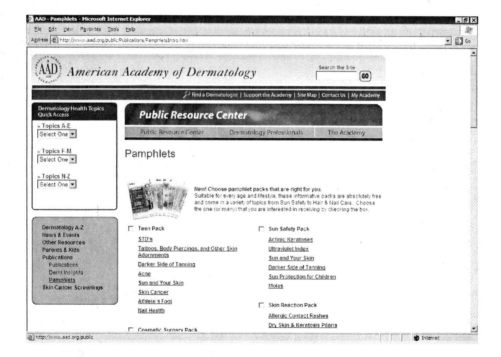

FIGURE 8.1. American Academy of Dermatology Home Page
<http://www.aad.org/public/Publications/PamphletsIntro.htm>

topics to dermatologic conditions. "News Releases" (select "News & Events," then "News Releases") also has useful information for patients.

American Society for Dermatologic Surgery
\<http://www.asds.net/Patients/FactSheets/patients-Fact_Sheet.html\>

The ASDS site offers information both for patients and members of the society. The "Fact Sheets" page links to fact sheets on procedures and techniques, definitions, and photographs. Procedures include treatment/ surgery for skin conditions such as acne scars, skin cancer, and tattoo removal, but also procedures such as hair restoration, liposuction, and eyelid surgery. Selecting "Your Skin Surgery Expert" connects you to information about training and services provided by dermatologic surgeons, along with summary information on procedures and photographs. "Find a Dermatologic Surgeon" helps locate a surgeon near you; links bring up member pages with contact information and procedures performed.

Facial Plastic Surgery Network
\<http://www.facialplasticsurgery.net\>

"The Facial Plastic Surgery Network is dedicated to helping you obtain solutions to your facial aesthetic concerns." This site is produced by Enhancement Media, a company that has a group of related sites on cosmetic surgery topics. The site is easy to navigate, with links to pages on "Facial Procedures," "Choosing a Surgeon," "Procedure FAQ," "Anesthesia Information," a photo gallery, chat groups and discussion forums, and more. A key page is "Facial Procedures," which has links to an extensive list of procedures (some of these are individually listed later in this chapter and also in Chapter 7, "Cosmetic Surgery of the Face, Head, and Neck"). About half of the procedures listed on this page are skin related. Information is similar to the site **Yes They're Fake!** which is also produced by the same company.

   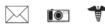

iEnhance—Facial Plastic Surgery
<http://www.ienhance.com/speciality/facial.asp>

Cosmetic procedures of the skin are included by iEnhance in their Facial Plastic Surgery page. Go directly to the URL (*sic*—speciality in URL), or begin at the general <http://www.ienhance.com> and select "Facial Plastic Surgery." This page has links to featured articles, archived articles, a photo gallery, a doctor locator, and specific surgical procedures. Select "Procedures" from this page, and then "Facial Plastic Surgery" to link to information on twenty-five to thirty facial plastic surgery procedures (see Figure 7.2 in Chapter 7), from dermabrasion and chemical peel to laser hair removal and Botox. Included are surgical procedures of the face (see Chapter 7) and hair transplantation (see Chapter 9).

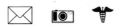

Yes They're Fake!—Facial Enhancement
<http://www.yestheyrefake.net/facial_plastic_surgery.html>

This candid site was created by a patient who has undergone cosmetic surgery. A majority of the specific procedures from the "Facial Enhancement" page are listed later in this chapter (or in Chapter 7, "Cosmetic Surgery of the Face, Head, and Neck") under the specific procedure, but it was not possible to list all (e.g., "Hyperpigmentation Removal," "Intense Pulsed Light," and "Obagi NuDerm System").

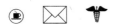

BOTULINUM TOXIN (BOTOX) INJECTIONS

Botulinum toxin (Botox) is a toxin that is injected into the skin to remove wrinkles and lines. Originally used to treat neurological disorders, Botox works by blocking nerve impulses, thus paralyzing muscles that can cause wrinkles. Botox is frequently injected into the forehead and lower face to reduce lines and wrinkles, and around the eyes to eliminate "crow's-feet." Botox is one of the most popular nonsurgical cosmetic procedures available today. Men account for about 11 percent of Botox injections, and both the ASPS and ASAPS list it as the top nonsurgical cosmetic procedure for men.

News reports and stories abound about "Botox parties," where people gather for injections. Be sure that the person administering Botox is a board-certified physician trained in this procedure.

2004 statistics:

ASAPS:	2,837,346	(311,916 in men)
ASPS:	2,992,607	(329,187 in men)

American Academy of Dermatology—Botulinum Toxin
<http://www.aad.org/public/Publications/pamphlets/Botulinum Toxin.htm>

This AAD pamphlet describes botulinum toxin (Botox), use of Botox for wrinkles, how it works, and side effects.

American Academy of Facial Plastic and Reconstructive Surgery— Botox Injections
<http://www.aafprs.org/media/media_resources/fact_botox.html>

AAFPRS provides brief information about Botox injections. The site cautions that Botox injections are a medical procedure and should be performed by a qualified facial plastic surgeon under appropriate conditions using sterile techniques.

American Society for Aesthetic Plastic Surgery—Botulinum Toxin Injections
<http://www.surgery.org/public/procedures-botoxing.php>

This ASAPS public page on Botox injections describes uses for botulinum toxin, the technique, benefits, and other considerations, along with an ASAPS position statement on the procedure.

American Society for Dermatologic Surgery—Botulinum Toxin Treatments
\<http://www.asds.net/Patients/FactSheets/patients-Fact_Sheet-botulinum_toxin.html\>

This ASDS fact sheet about Botox includes information about the toxin, how and where it is used, what to expect after treatment, and side effects.

American Society of Plastic Surgeons—Facial Rejuvenation (Botox)
\<http://www.plasticsurgery.org/public_education/procedures/Botox.cfm\>

The ASPS page on Botox provides a brief description about the injections and what the toxin does, but lists no side effects.

iEnhance—Botox® Cosmetic
\<http://www.ienhance.com/procedure/default.asp\>

From the "List of Procedures" select either "Plastic Surgery" or "Facial Plastic Surgery," then under "Head/Face" select "Botox Injections." The page includes basic information on the procedure, its benefits, risks, outcome, the ideal candidate for the procedure, and questions to ask your doctor.

MedlinePlus—Botox
<http://www.nlm.nih.gov/medlineplus/botox.html>

The Botox page on MedlinePlus (see Figure 8.2) directs you to quality information on Botox, including government and association sites. It's a good place to start.

U.S. Food and Drug Administration—Botox Cosmetic: A Look at Looking Good
<http://www.fda.gov/fdac/features/2002/402_botox.html>

This article, "Botox Cosmetic: A Look at Looking Good," was published in the July-August 2002 *FDA Consumer* magazine (see Figure 8.3). It explains how Botox works, mentions Botox "parties," and includes an FDA recommendation on use. Also available from the FDA is a Botox fact sheet at <http://www.fda.gov/womens/getthefacts/botox.html>.

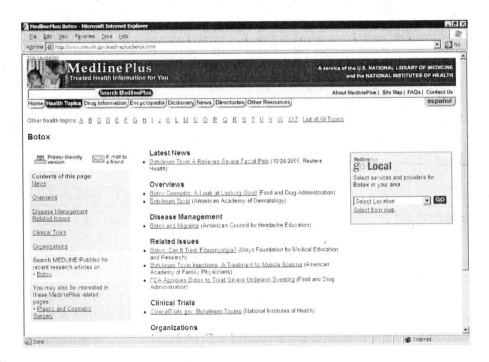

FIGURE 8.2. MedlinePlus—Botox
<http://www.nlm.nih.gov/medlineplus/botox.html>

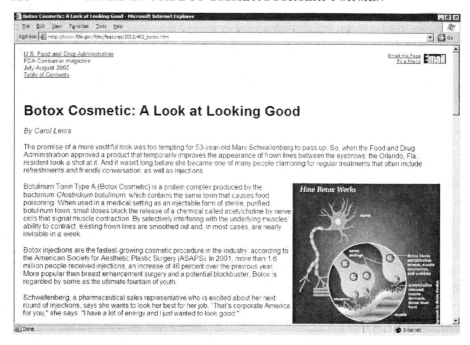

FIGURE 8.3. U.S. FDA—Botox Cosmetic
<http://www.fda.gov/fdac/features/2002/402_botox.html>

Yes They're Fake!—Botox
<http://www.yestheyrefake.net/botox.htm>

The page on Botox discusses what it is (a snake venom) and what it's used for, where it can be injected, what to expect, and risks, complications, and contraindications.

CELLULITE TREATMENT

Cellulite is the dimple-like fat that occurs primarily in women, frequently in the thighs, abdomen, and buttock areas. It can also occur in men. Treatments range from creams to liposuction, with varying levels of success.

2004 statistics:

ASAPS: 81,673   (767 in men)
ASPS: 44,569   (5,794 in men)

American Academy of Dermatology—Dermatologists Shed Light on Treatments for Cellulite
<http://www.aad.org/>

At the AAD site, do a site search for "cellulite" to find this archived press release, which describes cellulite and treatments—creams, mechanical massage, diet, and exercise. According to the AAD, there is no permanent solution.

American Skincare and Cellulite Expert Association
<http://www.ascea.org>

According to the Web site, "ASCEA is the largest and most innovative professional association serving the needs of hundreds of cellulite treatment centers in 20-plus countries." This site has information on cellulite anatomy (showing how women store fat differently than men), treatments, Endermologie (a trademarked system for "subdermal treatment for reducing cellulite"), and a directory of accredited centers. Although considered rare, men do have cellulite.

Yes They're Fake!—Cellulite Treatment
<http://www.yestheyrefake.net/cellulite_treatment_removal.htm>

Cellulite occurs in both women and men. The page reviews what cellulite is versus "normal" fat, treatment options (from Endermologie to liposuction to RejuveSkin), and discusses whether you are a candidate for cellulite removal, plus complications and risks. Also, check out another page on this site dedicated to "RejuveSkin Treatment for Cellulite," <http://www.yestheyrefake.net/rejuveskin_cellulite.htm>.

CHEMICAL PEELS

Chemical peels involve using a chemical solution on the surface of the skin to peel away the top layers of the skin. Factors such as the strength of the chemical and how long it is left on the skin will determine how many layers of skin are peeled away. Chemical peels are used to treat skin conditions such as wrinkles and imperfections in the skin (e.g., acne scars). Skin that is regenerated after chemical peeling is smoother and has less wrinkles than before. Chemical peels can be used with other procedures such as dermabrasion; this procedure is not a substitute for a facelift. Approximately 10 to 12 percent of chemical peels are performed on men.

2004 statistics:

ASAPS: 1,110,401   (133,124 in men)
ASPS: 1,090,523   (109,052 in men)

American Academy of Dermatology—Chemical Peeling
<http://www.aad.org/public/Publications/pamphlets/ChemicalPeeling.htm>

This AAD pamphlet describes what chemical peeling can do, how it is performed, what to expect after treatment, possible complications, and limitations of the procedure.

American Society for Aesthetic Plastic Surgery—Chemical Skin Peel (Light and Deep)
<http://www.surgery.org/public/procedures-chem_peel_light.php>
<http://www.surgery.org/public/procedures-chem_peel_deep.php>

The ASAPS has two public pages on chemical skin peels: one describes light to medium peels, the second reviews deep (phenol) peels. Each page describes uses for chemical peels, the technique, benefits, and other considerations. The deep peel page indicates what to expect after the procedure.

American Society for Dermatologic Surgery—Chemical Peeling
<http://www.asds.net/Patients/FactSheets/patients-Fact_Sheet-chem_peel.html>

This ASDS fact sheet about chemical peeling includes information about the procedure, why it's performed, and what to expect after treatment.

American Society of Plastic Surgeons—Chemical Peel
<http://www.plasticsurgery.org/public_education/procedures/ChemicalPeel.cfm>

The ASPS page on chemical peels provides fairly extensive information, including a general overview, preparing for a chemical peel, the procedure itself, and posttreatment. Three chemical solutions are described along with specific uses and considerations for each formula. Includes illustrations.

Facial Plastic Surgery Network—Chemical Peels
<http://www.facialplasticsurgery.net/chemical_peel.htm>

This page describes the chemical peeling procedure and options to the procedure, expectations, recovery, risks, and complications.

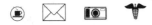

iEnhance—Chemical Peel
<http://www.ienhance.com/procedure/default.asp>

From the "List of Procedures" select either "Plastic Surgery" or "Facial Plastic Surgery," then under "Head/Face" select "Chemical Peel." Includes basic information such as surgical procedure, risks, postsurgical recovery, the ideal candidate for the procedure, and questions to ask your doctor.

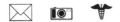

Yes They're Fake!—Chemical Peels
<http://www.yestheyrefake.net/chemical_peel.htm>

The page covers options for chemical peels, preoperative information, how the procedure is performed, the recovery, contraindications, and risks and complications.

COLLAGEN INJECTIONS

See under INJECTABLE FILLERS—Collagen Injections (in this chapter).

DERMABRASION

Dermabrasion is used to treat facial skin conditions such as acne scars, wrinkles, sun damage, and scars from accidents. The patient's skin is numbed and then the surgeon scrapes, or planes, the outer layer of skin. The new skin that forms under the treated area has a smoother appearance. Men account for approximately 13 to 14 percent of procedures.

2004 statistics:

ASAPS: 64,620* (8,534 in men)
ASPS: 54,018   (7,563 in men)

American Academy of Dermatology—Dermabrasion
<http://www.aad.org/public/Publications/pamphlets/
dermabrasion.htm>

This AAD pamphlet describes dermabrasion, indications for the procedure, how it is performed, possible complications, and limitations of the procedure.

---

*This number does not include miocrodermabrasion.

American Society for Dermatologic Surgery—Dermabrasion
<http://www.asds.net/Patients/FactSheets/patients-Fact_Sheet-dermabrasion.html>

This ASDS fact sheet about chemical peeling describes the procedure, when it should be used, and what to expect before, during, and after treatment.

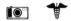

American Society of Plastic Surgeons—Dermabrasion (Skin Refinishing)
<http://www.plasticsurgery.org/public_education/procedures/Dermabrasion.cfm>

The ASPS page on dermabrasion (see Figure 8.4) provides fairly extensive information, including a general overview, alternative procedures, best candidates for the treatment, risks, preparing for dermabrasion, the surgery itself, and posttreatment.

Facial Plastic Surgery Network—Dermabrasion
<http://www.facialplasticsurgery.net/dermabrasion.htm>

This page includes a description of the procedure and discusses whether you are a candidate for the procedure, expectations, recovery, risks, and complications.

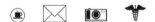

iEnhance—Dermabrasion
<http://www.ienhance.com/procedure/default.asp>

From the "List of Procedures" select either "Plastic Surgery" or "Facial Plastic Surgery," then under "Head/Face" select "Dermabrasion." The page includes basic information on the procedure, risks, postsurgical recovery, the ideal candidate for the procedure, and questions to ask your doctor.

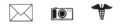

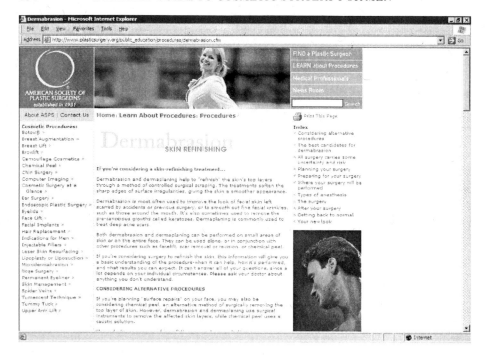

FIGURE 8.4. American Society of Plastic Surgeons—Dermabrasion
<http://www.plasticsurgery.org/public_education/procedures/dermabrasion.cfm>
©2004 American Society of Plastic Surgeons. All rights reserved. Learn more at
<www.plasticsurgery.org>.

Yes They're Fake!—Dermabrasion
<http://www.yestheyrefake.net/dermabrasion.htm>

The page covers whether you are a candidate for dermabrasion, preoperative information, how the procedure is performed, the recovery, and risks and complications.

ENDERMOLOGIE

See CELLULITE TREATMENT (in this chapter).

FAT INJECTIONS

See under INJECTABLE FILLERS—Fat Injections (in this chapter).

HAIR REPLACEMENT

See Chapter 9, "Hair Transplantation for Men."

HYALAFORM INJECTIONS

See under INJECTABLE FILLERS—Hyaluronic Acid (in this chapter).

HYALURONIC ACID INJECTIONS

See under INJECTABLE FILLERS—Hyaluronic Acid Injections (in this chapter).

INJECTABLE FILLERS

Injectable fillers are another form of cosmetic treatment used to make acne scars, wrinkles, and other facial skin imperfections less noticeable, and to restore a more youthful appearance to the skin. The most commonly used fillers are collagen and fat, and new fillers include Hylaform and Restylane; each of these fillers has specific subsections. When injected under the skin, these fillers eliminate wrinkles and make the skin look smoother. This treatment can be combined with other cosmetic procedures, such as facial resurfacing or a facelift. Botox, while an injectable, is a muscle paralyzer, not a filler; it is listed earlier in this chapter.

American Academy of Dermatology—Soft Tissue Fillers
<http://www.aad.org/public/Publications/pamphlets/
  SoftTissueFillers.htm>

This AAD page talks about what soft tissue fillers are and what they can do; briefly describes several types of fillers; and describes the procedure, risks, and treatment options.

American Society for Aesthetic Plastic Surgery—Injectables
<http://www.surgery.org/public/procedures-injectables.php>

This ASAPS public page on injectables describes techniques, uses, and benefits for botulinum toxin, collagen, fat, and hyaluronic acid injections.

American Society of Plastic Surgeons—Injectable Fillers
  (Improving Skin Texture)
<http://www.plasticsurgery.org/public_education/procedures/
  InjectableFillers.cfm>

This ASPS page (see Figure 8.5) discusses what fillers are used for, options to fillers, risks, and the procedure (with a focus on collagen and fat fillers).

Facial Plastic Surgery Network—Injectables: Fillers for Soft Tissue
  Augmentation
<http://www.facialplasticsurgery.net/injectable_fillers.htm>

This page on injectables links to five pages of augmentation materials, by category: "Temporary Injectables," "Permanent Injectable Micro-implants," "Injectable Bio-catalysts," "Injectable Bio-implants," and "Injectable Self-derivative Products."

 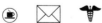

iEnhance—Skin Injection Treatments
<http://www.ienhance.com/procedure/default.asp>

From the "List of Procedures" select either "Plastic Surgery" or "Facial Plastic Surgery," then under "Head/Face" select "Skin Injection Treatments."

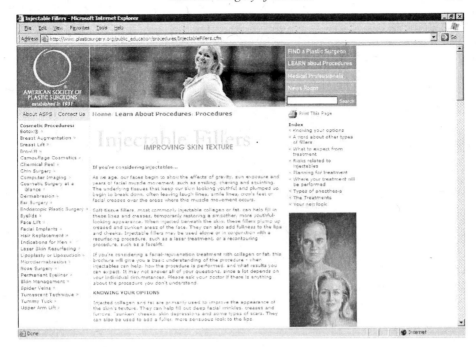

FIGURE 8.5. American Society of Plastic Surgeons—Injectable Fillers (Improving Skin Texture)
<http://www.plasticsurgery.org/public_education/procedures/InjectableFillers.cfm>
©2004 American Society of Plastic Surgeons. All rights reserved. Learn more at <www.plasticsurgery.org>.

The page includes benefits of the procedure, risks, postsurgical recovery, the ideal candidate for the procedure, and questions to ask your doctor. Injectables mentioned are: AlloDerm (including Cymetra), Botox, collagen, fat, silicone, and Restylane.

Collagen Injections

2004 statistics:

ASAPS: 785,448 (40,364 in men)
ASPS: 521,769 (31,306 in men)

American Academy of Cosmetic Surgery—Collagen
<http://www.cosmeticsurgery.org/Patients/collagen.asp>

The page contains basic information about the treatment.

American Society for Aesthetic Plastic Surgery—Collagen Injections
<http://www.surgery.org/public/procedures-collagen.php>

This ASAPS public page on collagen injections describes uses for collagen injections, the technique, benefits, and other considerations.

Fat Injections

2004 statistics:

ASAPS: 99,439 (5,908 in men)
ASPS: 56,377 (4,510 in men)

American Academy of Cosmetic Surgery—Fat Injections
<http://www.cosmeticsurgery.org/Patients/fatinjections.asp>

This page describes reasons for using fat injections, the procedure, and the possibility of storing fat for future use.

American Society for Aesthetic Plastic Surgery—Fat Injection
<http://www.surgery.org/public/procedures-fatinject.php>

This ASAPS public page describes uses for fat injections, the technique, benefits, and other considerations. This page was still available but not listed on the Procedures page; look for the page on Injectables. In the Photo Gallery, look under "Soft Tissue Fillers."

American Society for Dermatologic Surgery—Microlipoinjection (or Fat Transfer)
<http://www.asds.net/Patients/FactSheets/patients-Fact_Sheet-microlipoinjection.html>

This ASDS fact sheet about microlipoinjection describes the procedure and its uses.

Facial Plastic Surgery Network—Fat Grafting (Fat Transfer)
<http://www.facialplasticsurgery.net/fat_grafting.htm>

The fat grafting page describes the procedure, along with whether you are a candidate for the procedure, expectations, recovery, risks and complications, and more.

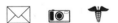

iEnhance—Fat Injections
<http://www.ienhance.com/procedure/default.asp>

From the "List of Procedures" select either "Plastic Surgery" or "Facial Plastic Surgery," then under "Head/Face" select "Fat Injections." The page includes basic information about the surgical procedure, benefits, risks, postsurgical recovery, the ideal candidate for the procedure, and questions to ask your doctor.

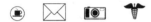

Yes They're Fake!—Fat Grafting
<http://www.yestheyrefake.net/fat_grafting.htm>

The page describes the procedure, whether you are a good candidate, expectations, the recovery, and risks and complications.

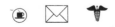

Hyaluronic Acid Injections (including Hylaform and Restylane)

American Academy of Cosmetic Surgery—Hylaform®
and Hylaform Plus®
<http://www.cosmeticsurgery.org/Patients/hylaform.asp>

The page on Hylaform contains basic information about this relatively new treatment (FDA approved in 2004).

American Academy of Cosmetic Surgery—Restylane™
<http://www.cosmeticsurgery.org/Patients/restylane.asp>

The page contains basic information about the treatment.

American Society for Dermatologic Surgery—Restylane®
(Hyaluronic Acid)
<http://asds-net.org/Media/PositionStatements/White_Paper-
Restylane.html>

The ASDS white paper on Restylane describes the product and its uses. Approved by the FDA in December 2003 for use in the United States, it has been used in Europe for about ten years. The ASDS also has several media releases available through its Media page.

iEnhance—Restylane®
<http://www.ienhance.com/procedure/default.asp>

From the "List of Procedures" select "Facial Plastic Surgery" and then "Restylane." The page includes basic information about the injectable filler, based on hyaluronic acid, that is used to reduce the signs of aging. Included is information about what to expect from the treatment, the ideal candidate, risks, and questions to ask your doctor.

U.S. Food and Drug Administration. Center for Devices and Radiological Health—New Device Approval. Hyalaform—P030032
<http://www.fda.gov/cdrh/mda/docs/p030032.html>

This page summarizes the approval process for Hylaform, a modified hylauronic acid derived from an avian source, how it works, how it is used, and how it should not be used. A link is available to the FDA posting of the summary of the safety and effectiveness of the product.

U.S. Food and Drug Administration. Center for Devices and Radiological Health—New Device Approval. Restylane™ Injectable Gel—P040024
<http://www.fda.gov/cdrh/mda/docs/p040024.html>

This page summarizes the approval process for Restylane, a nonanimal hyaluronic acid gel, how it works, how it is used, and how it should not be used. A link is available to the FDA posting of the summary of the safety and effectiveness of the product.

LASER HAIR REMOVAL

Laser hair removal is a popular new treatment for permanent removal of unwanted hair from the face or body. A low-energy laser is applied through the skin into the hair follicle, thus damaging the follicle and stopping hair growth.

2004 statistics:

ASAPS: 1,411,899 (196,847 in men)
ASPS: 573,970 (154,972 in men)

American Society for Aesthetic Plastic Surgery—Laser Hair Removal
<http://www.surgery.org/public/procedures-hairremove.php>

This ASAPS public page on hair removal contains information about this nonsurgical procedure, benefits, and other considerations. Laser hair removal is used on the face and other parts of the body.

American Society for Dermatologic Surgery—Laser Hair Removal
<http://www.asds.net/Patients/FactSheets/patients-Fact_Sheet-
 laser_hair_removal.html>

This ASDS fact sheet about laser hair removal includes information about hair growth, the laser hair removal procedure, types of lasers, and the advantages and limitations of laser hair removal.

iEnhance—Laser Hair Removal
<http://www.ienhance.com/procedure/default.asp>

From the "List of Procedures" select either "Plastic Surgery" or "Facial Plastic Surgery," then under "Head/Face" select "Laser Hair Removal." The page includes basic information on the procedure, risks, what to expect afterward, the ideal candidate for the procedure, and questions to ask your doctor.

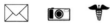

MayoClinic.com—Laser Hair Removal: Zapping Unwanted Hair
<http://www.mayoclinic.com/invoke.cfm?id=HQ00981>

Go directly to the URL, or go to the general Mayo site <http://www. mayoclinic.com> and do a site search for "laser hair removal." This page tells you how to prepare for the procedure and how it is performed. At the end, link to "Hair Removal 101: A Comparison of Different Techniques."

LASER SKIN RESURFACING

Laser skin resurfacing is used to remove wrinkles, scars, and areas of damaged skin. It can be used on the whole face, but is especially helpful in minimizing lines around the eyes ("crow's-feet") and mouth. Lasers can be more precise than chemical peels or dermabrasion. Laser resurfacing is often done in combination with another procedure such as eyelid surgery or a facelift.

2004 statistics:

ASAPS: 589,721 (69,427 in men)
ASPS: 164,451 (14,801 in men)

American Academy of Cosmetic Surgery—Laser Resurfacing
<http://www.cosmeticsurgery.org/Patients/laserskinresurfacing.asp>

This page contains brief information about laser resurfacing.

American Academy of Dermatology—Laser Resurfacing for Facial Skin Rejuvenation
<http://www.aad.org/public/Publications/pamphlets/ LaserResurfacingRejuv.htm>

This AAD pamphlet describes the procedure of laser resurfacing, types of lasers and what they are used for, what to expect during and after the treatment, and possible complications and limitations of the procedure.

American Society for Dermatologic Surgery—Laser Resurfacing
<http://www.asds.net/Patients/FactSheets/patients-Fact_Sheet- laser_resurfacing.html>

This ASDS fact sheet about laser resurfacing describes the procedure, why it's performed, types of lasers (more can be found under "Laser Applications"), what to expect during and after treatment, and side effects/ complications.

American Society of Plastic Surgeons—Laser Skin Resurfacing
<http://www.plasticsurgery.org/public_education/procedures/
  Laser-Skin-Resurfacing.cfm>

This ASPS page on laser skin resurfacing provides a brief description about the procedure and what it is used for, but lists no side effects. More extensive information is available from the "Reconstructive Procedures" list, which includes skin resurfacing, <http://www.plasticsurgery.org/public_education/procedures/SkinResurfacing.cfm>.

Facial Plastic Surgery Network—Laser Resurfacing & Laser
  Treatments
<http://www.facialplasticsurgery.net/laser_resurfacing.htm>

This page describes lasers and how they work, laser resurfacing and types of lasers, plus how laser resurfacing is performed and whether you are a good candidate, the recovery, and risks and complications. Also check out the page on "NLite Laser" <http://www.facialplasticsurgery.net/NLite.htm>.

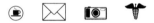

iEnhance—Laser Skin Resurfacing
<http://www.ienhance.com/procedure/default.asp>

From the "List of Procedures" select either "Plastic Surgery" or "Facial Plastic Surgery," then under "Head/Face" select "Laser Skin Resurfacing." The page includes basic information such as surgical procedure, types of lasers, risks, postsurgical recovery, the ideal candidate for the procedure, and questions to ask your doctor.

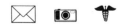

MayoClinic.com—Laser Resurfacing: Treatment for Younger Looking Skin
<http://www.mayoclinic.com/invoke.cfm?id=WO00008>

Go directly to the URL or go to the general Mayo site <http://www.mayoclinic.com> and do a site search for "laser resurfacing." The procedure is described along with how to prepare for the procedure, recovery information, complications and risks, and the need for real expectations.

Yes They're Fake!—Laser Treatments
<http://www.yestheyrefake.net/laser_resurfacing.htm>

The page describes lasers and how they work, laser resurfacing and types of lasers, plus how laser resurfacing is performed and whether you are a good candidate, the recovery, and risks and complications. Also check out the page on "NLite Laser," <http://yestheyrefake.net/NLite.htm>.

LASER TREATMENT OF SPIDER VEINS

This procedure removes spider veins using a laser. It is most frequently performed on spider veins of the face, as spider veins elsewhere on the body are normally removed with sclerotherapy.

2004 statistics:

ASAPS: 207,612 (9,858 in men)
ASPS: 103,460 (14,484 in men)

iEnhance—Laser Spider Vein Treatment
<http://www.ienhance.com/procedure/default.asp>

From the "List of Procedures" select either "Plastic Surgery" or "Facial Plastic Surgery," then under "Head/Face" or "Legs" select "Laser Spider

Vein Treatment." The page includes basic information such as surgical procedure, risks, postsurgical recovery, the ideal candidate for the procedure, and questions to ask your doctor.

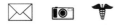

MICRODERMABRASION

Microdermabrasion is a nonsurgical treatment for fine lines and wrinkles in the face. The technique involves "brushing" of the face with crystals, which stimulates production of collagen and skin cells, resulting in a more youthful appearance.

2004 statistics:

ASAPS:	1,098,316	(99,221 in men)
ASPS:	858,867	(214,717 in men)

**American Society for Aesthetic Plastic Surgery—
Microdermabrasion**
<http://www.surgery.org/public/procedures-microderm.php>

This ASAPS public page on microdermabrasion, a nonsurgical cosmetic procedure, contains general information about the procedure, a description of the technique, benefits, and other considerations.

**American Society of Plastic Surgeons—Microdermabrasion
(Surface-Repair Treatments)**
**<http://www.plasticsurgery.org/public_education/procedures/
Microdermabrasion.cfm>**

This ASPS page on microdermabrasion provides a brief description about microdermabrasion and what the procedure is used for, but lists no side effects.

Facial Plastic Surgery Network—Microdermabrasion
<http://www.facialplasticsurgery.net/microdermabrasion.htm>

This page describes the microdermabrasion procedure, helps you decide whether you are a candidate for the procedure, and discusses expectations, recovery, risks and complications, and more.

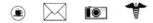

Yes They're Fake!—Microdermabrasion
<http://www.yestheyrefake.net/microdermabrasion.htm>

This page on microdermabrasion covers everything from whether you are a good candidate for this procedure and what to expect during and after the treatment, to expectations about the procedure and risks. Included is a discussion of machines used for microdermabrasion.

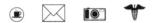

MICROPIGMENTATION (PERMANENT MAKEUP)

Micropigmentation has been given a number of names: cosmetic tattooing, dermapigmentation, and permanent makeup. This procedure has rapidly gained popularity for people who have allergies to cosmetics, have difficulty putting on makeup, or who want a permanent cosmetic enhancement.

American Academy of Dermatology—Tattoos, Body Piercings,
and Other Skin Adornments
<http://www.aad.org/public/Publications/PamphletsIntro.htm>

This page describes five types of tattoos, complications and removal of tattoos; body piercing, complications and removal of piercings; and other types of skin adornments.

**American Society for Aesthetic Plastic Surgery—
 Micropigmentation
<http://www.surgery.org/public/procedures-micropigment.php>**

This ASAPS public page on micropigmentation contains general information about the procedure, benefits, and other considerations.

**American Society of Plastic Surgeons—Permanent Eyeliner
<http://www.plasticsurgery.org/public_education/procedures/
 Permanent-Eyeliner.cfm>**

This ASPS page on permanent eyeliner is a brief description about micropigmentation, the procedure used to create permanent makeup. Benefits, but no side effects, are listed.

**Facial Plastic Surgery Network—Micropigmentation (Permanent
 Make Up)
<http://www.facialplasticsurgery.net/micropigmentation.htm>**

This page describes the micropigmentation procedure, indicates body locations where it is done, and talks about the need to check the technician's background, expectations, recovery, risks and complications, and more.

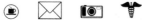

**iEnhance—Permanent Cosmetics
<http://www.ienhance.com/procedure/default.asp>**

From the "List of Procedures" select either "Plastic Surgery" or "Facial Plastic Surgery," then under "Head/Face" select "Permanent Cosmetics." The page includes basic information such as surgical procedure, risks, postsurgical recovery, the ideal candidate for the procedure, and questions to ask your doctor.

Yes They're Fake!—Micropigmentation
<http://www.yestheyrefake.net/micropigmentation.html>

The page on micropigmentation talks about what dermagraphics is, training and certifications for technicians, how the procedure is done, and areas where it is done. It is made clear that micropigmentation is tattooing.

   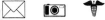

PERMANENT COSMETICS

See MICROPIGMENTATION (PERMANENT MAKEUP) (in this chapter).

RESTYLANE INJECTIONS

See under INJECTABLE FILLERS—Hyaluronic Acid Injections (in this chapter).

SCARS/SCAR REVISION

Scars can be caused by accidents, burns, or surgery. With scar revision, a variety of treatments or surgery can be used to remove, relocate, or make a scar less visible.

2004 statistics:

ASPS: 187,386 (no gender breakdown)

American Academy of Dermatology—What is a Scar
<http://www.aad.org/public/Publications/pamphlets/WhatisaScar.htm>

This AAD pamphlet describes what can be done for scars; treatments range from surgical scar revision and dermabrasion to laser resurfacing and chemical peels; an extensive list of other possible treatments is given.

American Academy of Facial Plastic and Reconstructive Surgery— Understanding Facial Scar Treatment
<http://www.aafprs.org/patient/procedures/facial_scar.html>

The AAFPRS site (see Figure 8.6) discusses making the decision to have skin resurfacing, types of procedures (Z-plasty, dermabrasion), and what to expect postsurgery; the focus is on scar revision of the face. Before/after illustrations are included.

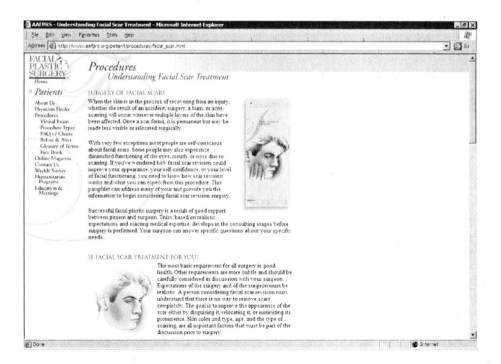

FIGURE 8.6. American Academy of Facial Plastic and Reconstructive Surgery— Understanding Facial Scar Treatment
<http://www.aafprs.org/patient/procedures/facial_scar.html>
Reprinted with permission of American Academy of Facial Plastic and Reconstructive Surgery.

American Society of Plastic Surgeons—Scar Revision
<http://www.plasticsurgery.org/public_education/procedures/ ScarRevision.cfm>

The ASPS page on scar revision describes why you might consider this procedure, types of scars, risks of surgery, types of surgical procedures (Z-plasty, skin grafting, and flap surgery), and postsurgical information.

Facial Plastic Surgery Network—Scar Revision & Keloid Prevention
<http://www.facialplasticsurgery.net/scar_revision.htm>

This page is similar to Yes They're Fake! and describes the scar revision procedure, whether you would make a good candidate, expectations, recovery, risks and complications, and more.

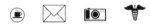

iEnhance—Scar Revision/Scar Repair
<http://www.ienhance.com/procedure/default.asp>

From the "List of Procedures" select either "Plastic Surgery" or "Facial Plastic Surgery," then under "Head/Face" select "Scar Revision/Scar Repair." The page includes basic information on the benefits of this surgery, options for surgical procedure, risks, postsurgical recovery, the ideal candidate for the procedure, and questions to ask your doctor. Procedures for scar revision include collagen injections, dermabrasion, laser skin resurfacing, punch grafting, tissue expansion, Z-plasty, and more.

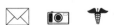

Yes They're Fake!—Scar Revision
<http://www.yestheyrefake.net/scar_revision.htm>

Go directly to the URL, or go to the main page <http://www.yestheyre fake.net>, select "Facial Procedures," and then "Scar Revision." The page describes scar revision, whether you are a candidate for the procedure, preoperative information, how the procedure is performed, the recovery, contraindications, and risks and complications.

SCLEROTHERAPY

Spider veins (more technically called telangiectasias), are those small red, purple, or blue veins that appear on the thigh or lower leg, but can be located elsewhere on the body. They are broken veins or capillaries that can be removed without causing harm.

Sclerotherapy is the most frequently used treatment for spider veins. A sclerosing solution (saline—salt solution) is injected into the vein with a small needle; multiple injections are needed for each session. The solution causes the vein to collapse and gradually disappear. Spider veins in the facial area are usually treated with lasers instead of sclerotherapy.

2004 statistics:

ASAPS: 487,987 (8,827 in men)
ASPS: 544,898 (5,449 in men)

American Academy of Cosmetic Surgery—Sclerotherapy
<http://www.cosmeticsurgery.org/Patients/sclerotherapy.asp>

The page contains a basic statement about sclerotherapy.

American Academy of Dermatology—Spider Vein, Varicose Vein Therapy
<http://www.aad.org/public/Publications/pamphlets/SpiderVein.htm>

This AAD pamphlet describes spider veins, their prevention, and treatment. The primary treatment described in this pamphlet is sclerotherapy, although laser treatment is among several additional procedures mentioned.

American Society for Aesthetic Plastic Surgery—Sclerotherapy
<http://www.surgery.org/public/procedures-sclerotherapy.php>

The ASAPS page on sclerotherapy, the treatment for spider veins, describes the technique, benefits, and other considerations.

American Society for Dermatologic Surgery—Spider and Varicose Veins
<http://www.asds.net/Patients/FactSheets/patients-Fact_Sheet-veins.html>

This ASDS fact sheet (see Figure 8.7) talks about spider and varicose veins and then focuses on sclerotherapy as the "gold standard" treatment for

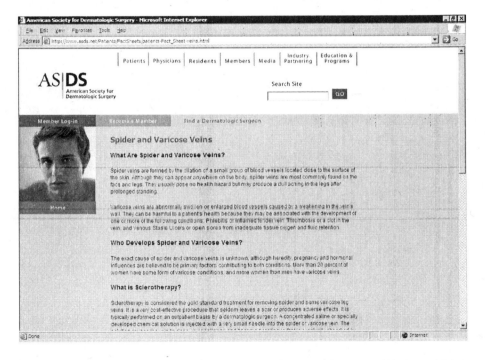

FIGURE 8.7. American Society for Dermatologic Surgery—Spider and Varicose Veins <http://www.asds.net/Patients/FactSheets/patients-Fact_Sheet-veins.html> Reprinted with permission of American Society for Dermatologic Surgery.

spider veins. Other treatments (laser surgery, electrodesiccation, surgical ligation and stripping, and ambulatory phlebectomy) are mentioned.

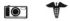

American Society of Plastic Surgeons—Sclerotherapy (Spider Veins)
<http://www.plasticsurgery.org/public_education/procedures/Sclerotherapy.cfm>

This ASPS page on spider veins (sclerotherapy) includes a description of spider veins, candidates for surgery, a description of the treatment, along with risks and what to expect from the procedure.

iEnhance—Spider Vein Treatment (Sclerotherapy)
<http://www.ienhance.com/procedure/default.asp>

From the "List of Procedures" select "Plastic Surgery," then under "Legs" select "Spider Vein Treatment (Sclerotherapy)." The page includes basic information about spider veins, but focuses on sclerotherapy, the primary surgical procedure for spider veins, including risks, postsurgical recovery, the ideal candidate for the procedure, and questions to ask your doctor. A link is available to "laser treatment," which can also be used for spider veins.

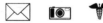

SKIN MANAGEMENT

See BOTULINUM (BOTOX) TOXIN, CHEMICAL PEELS, DERMABRASION, INJECTABLE FILLERS, LASER SKIN RESURFACING, SKIN RESURFACING, and WRINKLE TREATMENT (all in this chapter).

SKIN RESURFACING

Skin resurfacing smooths and refinishes the skin by removing blemishes, fine wrinkles, and other surface irregularities, resulting in a younger look. Methods used for skin resurfacing include chemical peels, derma-brasion, and laser resurfacing, each of which has its own section in this chapter. This section includes sites that review skin resurfacing as a whole. *See also* CHEMICAL PEELS, DERMABRASION, and LASER SKIN RESURFAC-ING (in this chapter).

American Academy of Facial Plastic and Reconstructive Surgery—Understanding Skin Resurfacing
<http://www.aafprs.org/patient/procedures/resurfacing.html>

The AAFPRS site discusses the decision to have skin resurfacing, types of procedures (chemical peels, dermabrasion, laser surgery), and what to expect postsurgery; includes before/after illustrations.

American Society for Aesthetic Plastic Surgery—Skin Resurfacing
<http://www.surgery.org/public/procedures-skinresurface.php>

This ASAPS public page on skin resurfacing, a technique used primar-ily on the face, leads to additional pages containing information about the surgical procedure, risks, before and after surgery, and more. This is one of the better sites available about skin resurfacing.

American Society of Plastic Surgeons—Skin Resurfacing (Lasers in Plastic Surgery)
<http://www.plasticsurgery.org/public_education/procedures/ SkinResurfacing.cfm>

Although this ASPS page is listed as skin resurfacing, it is specifically focused on laser skin resurfacing. Included is information about what the treatment is used for, a description of the procedure, best candidates for the procedure, risks, and what to expect from the procedure. The ASPS also has a separate page for Laser Skin Resurfacing.

SOFT TISSUE FILLERS

See INJECTABLE FILLERS (in this chapter).

SPIDER VEINS

See LASER TREATMENT OF SPIDER VEINS AND SCLEROTHERAPY (both in this chapter).

TATTOO REMOVAL

Tattoos can be removed with laser surgery, dermabrasion, or surgically; your physician will recommend the best treatment. *See also* DERMABRASION, LASER SKIN RESURFACING, and MICROPIGMENTATION (all in this chapter).

American Society for Dermatologic Surgery—Tattoo Removal
<http://www.asds.net/Patients/FactSheets/patients-Fact_Sheet-tattoo_removal.html>

The ASDS fact sheet about tattoo removal includes information about tattoos, the procedures used to remove them (laser surgery, dermabrasion, surgical excision), and side effect/complication information.

Facial Plastic Surgery Network—Tattoo Removal
<http://www.facialplasticsurgery.net/tattoo_removal.htm>

This page (see Figure 8.8) covers the tattoo removal process, whether you are a candidate for the procedure, various options for tattoo removal, recovery, risks and complications, and more.

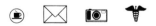

iEnhance—Tattoo Removal
<http://www.ienhance.com/procedure/default.asp>

From the "List of Procedures" select either "Plastic Surgery" or "Facial Plastic Surgery," then under "Head/Face" select "Tattoo Removal." The page

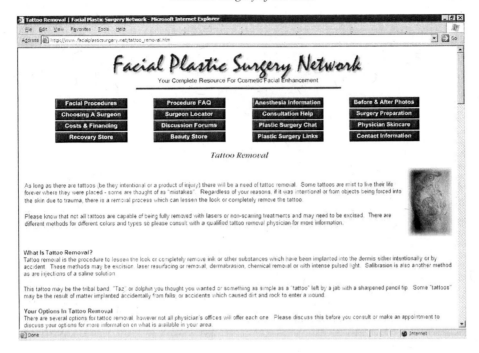

FIGURE 8.8. Facial Plastic Surgery Network—Tattoo Removal
<http://www.facialplasticsurgery.net/tattoo_removal.htm>
Reprinted with permission of Enhancement Media.

includes basic information such as surgical procedure (laser removal), risks, postsurgical recovery, the ideal candidate for the procedure, and questions to ask your doctor.

Yes They're Fake!—Tattoo Removal
<http://www.yestheyrefake.net/tattoo_removal.html>

The page covers options in tattoo removal, preoperative information, how the procedure is performed, the recovery, contraindications, and risks and complications.

THERMAGE

Thermage, or ThermaLift, is a new treatment for tightening aging skin. Since there is no incision, there are no scars or downtime involved. This treatment is also called a "nonsurgical facelift."

American Academy of Cosmetic Surgery—Thermage
<http://www.cosmeticsurgery.org/Patients/
thermagenonsurgicalfacelift.asp>

The page describes Thermage and how it works, possible need for pain relievers, and also posttreatment information.

Yes They're Fake!—Thermacool Thermoplasty
<http://www.yestheyrefake.net/thermacool_thermage.htm>

The page describes the procedure (heating the skin by radio-frequency waves to tighten the collagen in your skin), areas that can be treated, and everything from preparing for the treatment through recovery and possible complications. Average prices are given, and links are available to other resources.

WRINKLE TREATMENT

Wrinkles develop over time and are primarily a result of aging. The sites included in this section overview the various treatments for aging skin, from over-the-counter creams and lotions to Botox, skin resurfacing, and dermabrasion (see cross-references). *See also* other procedures such as BOTULINUM (BOTOX) TOXIN, CHEMICAL PEELS, DERMABRASION, INJECT-ABLE FILLERS, and LASER SKIN RESURFACING (all in this chapter).

American Academy of Dermatology—Facial Skin Rejuvenation
<http://www.aad.org/public/Publications/pamphlets/
FacialSkinRejuvenation.htm>

This AAD pamphlet describes the general process of aging skin and procedures that might be used for rejuvenation, including topical products, fillers, chemical peels, dermabrasion, laser resurfacing, liposuction, and surgery. Treatment of each topic is brief, as this is an overview document. A related pamphlet to check out at this site is "Mature Skin," <http://www. aad.org/public/Publications/pamphlets/MatureSkin.htm>.

American Academy of Facial Plastic and Reconstructive Surgery— Understanding Wrinkle Treatment
<http://www.aafprs.org/patient/procedures/wrinkles.html>

This AAFPRS page describes the various treatments for removing wrinkles from the face (including Botox, injectable collagen, and synthetic implants); it also discusses which treatment to choose, or combining these treatments with another surgical procedure, and what to expect after the treatment. Includes before/after illustrations.

American Society of Plastic Surgeons—Skin Management (Surface- Repair Treatments)
<http://www.plasticsurgery.org/public_education/procedures/
SkinManagement.cfm>

The ASPS page on skin management covers the nonsurgical procedures of Retin-A and glycolic acid treatments. Included is a description of these two treatments, best candidates for the treatments, reactions/side effects, and posttreatment information.

Yes They're Fake!—Wrinkles
<http://www.yestheyrefake.net/wrinkle_improvement.html>

This page on wrinkles covers everything from over-the-counter lotions and creams to implants, Botox, chemical peels, and microdermabrasion.

Chapter 9

Hair Transplantation for Men

Hair loss has been a concern of men since ancient times. In ancient Egypt and Greece, various mixtures were unsuccessfully used to try to regrow hair. Later, in the 1600s and 1700s, wigs became popular in Europe. Although they were considered a fashion statement, wigs also served to conceal hair loss.[1]

Hair transplantation, a relatively new treatment for hair loss, was pioneered during World War II, but only came into use as a cosmetic procedure in the United States in the late 1950s/early 1960s. Through the 1970s, early hair transplantation used large "punch" grafts of hair taken from the back and sides of the head, and was inserted as "plugs" in rows, hence the term "corn rows." These large punch grafts were replaced with smaller, mini- and micrografts in the 1980s. Minigrafts have about four to eight hairs; micrografts have one to three hairs. Used in combination, mini- and micrografts produced a more natural look. By the 1990s, follicular unit hair transplantation (FUT) had become the gold standard. FUT uses naturally occurring follicular unit groupings of one to four hairs. The procedure has been further refined as follicular unit extraction (FUE), in which follicles are extracted and transplanted individually.[2]

According to the American Society of Plastic Surgeons, hair transplantation was the second most popular cosmetic surgical procedure for men in 2004, with 43,054 procedures, or 88 percent of the 48,925 hair transplants performed by its member physicians; this represented a 54 percent increase in the number of men having hair transplants in 2004 (43,054) versus 2003 (27,985). The American Society for Aesthetic Plastic Surgery statistics for 2004 show that hair transplantation was the fifth most popular

Internet Guide to Cosmetic Surgery for Men
© 2006 by The Haworth Press, Inc. All rights reserved.
doi:10.1300/5854_10

surgical procedure for men, with 19,503 procedures reported, or 85 percent of the total 22,890 hair transplantations reported to the ASAPS.

In addition to hair transplantation, hair restoration treatments range from the use of drugs to wigs and hairpieces. Two medications are now approved by the FDA for treating hair loss. Minoxidil (Rogaine) and finasteride (Propecia, Proscar) have been shown to stimulate hair growth and reverse hair loss. Your choice of a treatment—surgical or nonsurgical—will be determined by your personal preference and goals for how you want to look and daily time that you have available to treat your hair loss. Over-the-counter hair medications must be administered daily; if discontinued, hair loss will resume. In addition, some maintenance is required for wigs and hairpieces. Because hair transplantation is viewed as the most effective cosmetic procedure for hair loss, it is the focus of this chapter; however, some sites cover both surgical and nonsurgical methods of treating hair loss.

Many of the clinics that perform hair transplantation procedures utilize technicians and lay people; physicians may be used only to perform occasional surgical procedures. You should be aware that there is no ABMS board certification for hair transplantation. Instead, you can expect your surgeon to be board certified in a variety of specialties, from plastic surgery to dermatology. A board certified physician who specializes in liposuction and body contouring but also performs occasional hair transplantation may not be the proper specialist for you.

A specialty organization, the American Board of Hair Restoration Surgery (ABHRS), was founded in 1996 by a small group of physicians who specialized in hair transplantation. In response to an invitation by the American Hair Loss Council, representatives from the American Academy of Cosmetic Surgery, International Society of Hair Restoration, American Academy of Facial Plastic and Reconstructive Surgery, and American Society of Dermatologic Surgery met and organized the ABHRS "to act for the benefit of the public to establish specialty standards and to examine surgeons' skill, knowledge and aesthetic judgment in the field of hair restoration surgery." The number of physicians certified by this organization remains small.

If you decide that hair transplantation is the right decision for you, you should look not only at the doctor's credentials, but his or her experience in hair transplantation. For instance, how many transplants does he or she perform per year; how long has he or she been performing transplants; and, is it the primary procedure that he or she performs? Ask to see examples of the doctor's work. Your physician should be willing to answer all of these questions to help you make your decision.

The Internet is overloaded with sites about hair loss—especially "miracle" cures proclaiming to stop hair loss, alternative forms of treatments, and special products. The sources listed represent carefully selected sites for you to locate information about hair transplantation. These include noncommercial sites such as organizations, associations, and government sites, plus commercial sites that have useful information related to hair restoration. The purpose of most hair restoration commercial sites is to introduce you to their services, i.e., to get you to contact them and make an appointment. However, many of these sites have excellent information, whether or not you choose to use the doctors/services listed on their site. This select list includes examples of private practices, group practices, and physician-locator services. Listing of a commercial site is not an endorsement of products, "locator" services, or physicians. Rather, these commercial sites were selected for one of two reasons: the site has a large amount of quality information about hair loss and/or hair transplantation, or the Web site is well done and subscribes to the HONcode principles.

HAIR TRANSPLANTATION SITES

American Academy of Dermatology—Hair Restoration
<http://www.aad.org/public/Publications/pamphlets/
HairRestoration.htm>

The AAD page on hair restoration offers basic information about normal hair growth, cause and types of hair loss, hair transplantation and other surgical options, and results to expect following surgery. The "Find a Dermatologist" link allows you to locate a board-certified dermatologist near you, but keep in mind that the physician may specialize in areas other than hair transplantation. From the "Dermatology Health Topics" link on the left, select "H" and find additional information, including a pamphlet on "Hair Loss," <http://www.aad.org/public/Publications/pamphlets/HairLoss.htm>, and "Alopecia Areata" <http://www.aad.org/public/Publications/pamphlets/AlopeciaAreata>.

American Academy of Facial Plastic and Reconstructive Surgery— Understanding Hair Replacement Surgery
<http://www.aafprs.org/patient/procedures/hair_replace.html>

The AAFPRS page (see Figure 9.1) has basic information about hair loss and hair replacement surgery, including making the decision to have surgery, information about the procedure, and what to expect after surgery. The physician finder has an extensive list of board certified physicians, but keep in mind that the surgeon may specialize in areas other than hair transplantation.

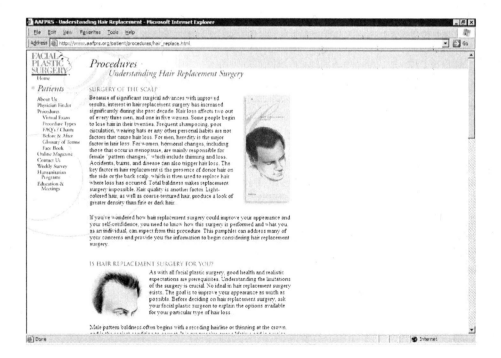

FIGURE 9.1. American Academy of Facial Plastic and Reconstructive Surgery— Understanding Hair Replacement Surgery
<http://www.aafprs.org/patient/procedures/hair_replace.html>
Reprinted with permission of American Academy of Facial Plastic and Reconstructive Surgery.

American Board of Hair Restoration Surgery
<http://www.abhrs.com>

The American Board of Hair Restoration Surgery (ABHRS) was founded in 1996. This site contains a "Directory of Diplomates," searchable by state and physician name, of physicians certified by the ABHRS. The list of certified physicians is extremely small. The section, "Application Process," includes certification requirements.

American Hair Loss Council
<http://www.ahlc.org>

The American Hair Loss Council, "the nation's only unbiased, not-for-profit agency," is composed of professionals and companies interested in treatment for hair loss, from manufacturers, cosmetologists, and barbers to dermatologists. The AHLC certifies nonphysician hair-loss specialists. The site includes nonbiased information about both surgical and non-surgical treatments and has a "Find a Specialist Near You," which is a membership directory searchable by state.

American Society for Aesthetic Plastic Surgery—Hair Transplantation
<http://surgery.org/public/procedures-hairtrans.php>

The ASAPS procedure page on hair transplantation covers basic hair transplant techniques, benefits, and other considerations. The "Find a Surgeon" feature allows you to locate a surgeon either inside or outside the United States, but keep in mind that the surgeon may not specialize in hair transplantation.

American Society for Dermatologic Surgery—Hair Restoration Treatments
<http://www.asds.net/Patients/FactSheets/patients-Fact_Sheet-hair_rest.html>

The ASDS fact sheet has general information about hair restoration, including surgical and nonsurgical techniques. "Find a Dermatologic Surgeon" links to an extensive list of dermatology certified surgeons, specialists in all areas of dermatologic surgery, and also allows you to limit your search to surgeons who perform hair transplantation.

American Society of Plastic Surgeons—Hair Replacement
<http://www.plasticsurgery.org/public_education/procedures/HairReplacement.cfm>

The ASPS public information page on hair replacement includes "best candidates" for hair replacement, a description of the surgery, risks, recovery after the surgery, and before/after illustrations. "Find a Plastic Surgeon" allows you to locate an ASPS member near you (not specific to hair transplants); you can look for either a cosmetic or reconstructive surgeon.

eMedicine—Hair Replacement Surgery/Hair Transplantation
<http://www.emedicine.com>

The eMedicine site is comprised of evidence-based articles on over 7,000 diseases. The content of eMedicine articles is at the professional level, so users of this site must be prepared for a more technical, medical approach than at other sites; however, the consumer version (eMedicineHealth) contains nothing about hair transplantation. Articles are "grouped" by medical specialty/subspecialty, and unfortunately, hair loss/disorders and hair transplantation articles are located in several sections, including "dermatology > surgical," "plastic surgery > hair," and "otolaryngology and facial plastic surgery > cosmetic surgery." Therefore, your best approach is to use the "Search" feature on the home page, entering simply the word "hair" (using hair transplantation actually misses one key article). Scroll through the articles (approximately 100) to find those relevant to you. You may also go to specific hair transplantation articles using the URLs listed here:

"Hair Transplantation"
<http://www.emedicine.com/derm/topic529.htm>
"Hair Graft Transplantation for Baldness"
<http://www.emedicine.com/ent/topic107.htm>
"Hair Replacement Surgery, Hair Transplantation"
<http://www.emedicine.com/plastic/topic61.htm>
"Hair Transplantation: Follicular Unit Transplant Method"
<http://www.emedicine.com/derm/topic559.htm>

In addition to the transplantation articles, consider also reading about related topics found in your search for "Hair," such as "Androgenetic Alopecia" and "Alopecia Areata." This site subscribes to the HONcode principles.

Hair Loss Learning Center
<http://www.regrowhair.com>

"The Hair Loss Learning Center is sponsored by the Coalition of independent Hair Restoration Physicians who believe that the best patient is an educated patient." The Coalition is a small group of prescreened physicians running independent practices, offering both surgical and nonsurgical treatments; membership is based on a "high level of ethics, skill, and the quality of their patient results," although more specific criteria are not listed. The site offers information on causes and the psychology of hair loss, the history of hair loss and treatments from ancient times to today's medications, follicular unit transplants, before-and-after photos, and a multimedia center with videos and animations. Links go to primarily commercial sites.

Hair Loss Patient Guide
<http://www.hairlosspatientguide.com>

This site has everything, from "All About Hair," causes of hair loss, and psychology of hair loss, to medical and surgical treatments, the transplant procedure, "Follicular Unit Hair Transplantation," and "Post Operation." Only an e-mail address is given for contact information; however, many of the pages are provided courtesy of the Physician's Hair Transplant Institute and clicking on that link takes you to the site of a hair transplant group, International Hair Transplant Institute (which is listed separately in this chapter).

Hair Loss Research
<http://www.hairlossresearch.com>

This site is a compilation of fairly technical articles about hair loss and hair transplantation, along with a collection of links to other sites, including links to physicians' medical practices/institutes. Examples of articles include "Hair Transplantation for Men With Advanced Degrees of Hair Loss" and "State of the Art Surgical Technique: Follicular Unit Hair Grafting," both by Dr. Jeffrey S. Epstein, a physician in private practice in Miami, Florida; "Creating a Natural Hairline" and "Follicular Unit Grafts vs. Small Mini Grafts," both by Dr. Ron Shapiro, a physician with a clinic in Minneapolis, Minnesota. Over ten physicians are listed as contributors to this site. All of the articles are technical but provide extensive, descriptive information not included on most other Internet sites.

Hair Loss Scams!
<http://www.hairlossscams.com>

This site, made available by DermMatch, Inc. (makers of DermMatch Topical Shading, one of the recommended products on this site), offers ways to spot a hair-loss scam and government agencies to contact about scams (e.g., FDA and FTC), with links included. Hair loss resources (books, Web sites, professional organizations) are also given. Keep in mind that even this site is not free of bias because of its commercial sponsorship.

Hair Loss Specialists
<http://www.hairlossspecialists.com>

This site has extensive information about hair loss, including causes of hair loss, differences between hair loss in women and men, treatment options, transplant surgery, a photo gallery, FAQs, and more. Choose "For Men" for specific information related to men (close the annoying pop-up window to see specific choices on the men's page). The "Find Hair Transplant Doctor" feature locates nationwide offices of Medical Hair Restoration, a private company, so this site is included for the information, rather than as a physician locator. The hair loss forums have postings from others who are also losing hair.

Hair Transplant Adviser
<http://www.hairtransplantadviser.org>

Despite this being listed as an organization (.org), it is a private site. The goal of the site is to help you "make the best possible choices in dealing with your hair loss." In addition to basic information on hair loss (including an excellent history) and hair transplantation, the site offers advice about realistic expectations, finding quality care, and tries to dispel some myths about hair transplantation. Follicular unit transplantation is emphasized as the preferred transplant method. Much of the content on this site is provided courtesy of the New Hair Institute (see separate listing in this chapter). A strength of the site is an extensive list of links. The International Alliance of Hair Restoration Surgeons is used as the physician-locator service (see separate listing in this chapter).

Hair Transplant Medical
<http://www.hairtransplantmedical.com>

This site has everything from the basics of hair growth and hair loss to treatments (e.g., medications, hair transplantation, alternative therapies). "Hair Transplant 101" includes "What is a Hair Transplant?" "Are you a Candidate?" and "Questions to ask your doctor," while "Beyond the Basics" has more in-depth topics such as "Bad Hair Transplants—Repair" and "When to be Suspicious." The site uses the International Alliance of Hair Restoration Surgeons as its physician-locator service, searchable by physician or state (of limited use because of small number of physicians). The site also includes article reprints from professional journals. Links to other sites provide additional resources. Although "Hair Transplant Medical is a consumer organization," it is, in fact, a physician-locator site that also provides consumer information. A drawback to this site is that its site "owner" could not be identified, other than the comment, "Please note that I am not a doctor, so I cannot provide you any advice for your hair loss," plus an e-mail address. The site suffers from multiple typographical errors.

Hair Transplant Network
<http://www.hairtransplantnetwork.com>

The Hair Transplant Network bills itself as the "#1 site for advice and top surgeons." It was created "by and for potential patients." The site offers a variety of information on hair transplantation in general, including basic information on hair restoration and transplantation, hair transplant articles (research library), "Best Hair Transplantation Procedure" (micro-follicular-unit hair transplantation), nonsurgical treatment, an extensive collection of before and after photos, and physician referral (members of the Coalition of Independent Hair Restoration Physicians are indicated). The site offers other features such as a discussion group, FAQs, a multimedia learning center, and "Find a 'Hair Loss Mentor.'"

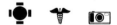

International Alliance of Hair Restoration Surgeons
<http://www.iahrs.org>

The IAHRS "is a consumer organization that selectively screens skilled and ethical hair transplant surgeons." This site includes the organization's mission, code of ethics, misconduct information and FAQs, along with members and a "Find a Doctor" service, plus a service to inquire about credentials of the doctor who performed your hair transplantation. Links are available to members' Web sites. This is a small, but growing organization in a field that does not have "official" board certification. Members of this organization must perform follicular unit hair transplantations, "prove their surgical skill and artistic ability," and "agree to impromptu inspections of their surgical facilities."

International Hair Transplant Institute
<http://www.forhair.com>

This is the site of the hair transplant group of Dr. John P. Cole, who heads a group that operates multiple sites in the United States and affiliate sites in Europe. The site contains information about the transplant procedure, discussion forums, a "live chat" link, and a patient guide (eighty-one-page PDF download) on hair restoration. This site contains contact information for prospective patients of this transplant group practice.

International Society of Hair Restoration Surgery
<http://www.ishrs.org>

The ISHRS is a "non-profit voluntary organization of over 700 hair restoration doctors specializing in hair loss." The mission of the society is "to advance the art and science of hair restoration by licensed, experienced physicians." Select "For Patients" to locate a wealth of information on the reasons for hair loss and both surgical and nonsurgical treatments of hair loss. "Common Questions About Hair Restoration" (FAQs); "Hair Loss Patient Stories"; and "Articles & Info" (scientific/medical articles about specialized topics) are available. The site contains information to help you select the right treatment along with excellent tips on selecting a doctor (e.g., checking credentials and training, experience, and comfort level). Also included is the "Find a Doctor" to help you locate a member of ISHRS near you; the listing includes about 700 specialists worldwide. In addition to address and phone information, many of the doctor profiles include e-mail addresses and Web sites for further information. The ISHRS site should be among the first that you visit when looking for basic hair transplantation information.

Medem Medical Library—Male Pattern Baldness (American Medical Association)
<http://www.medem.com>

Medem is "the nation's premier physician-patient communications network." It was created by seven leading medical associations and is now supported by more than forty national and state medical associations. Go to medem.com and then type baldness in the search box to locate the page on "Male Pattern Baldness," which is provided by the American Medical Association. The page describes the condition, causes of male-pattern baldness, describes other types of hair loss and diagnosis of the cause, and then describes medical (drug, surgical, and cosmetic) treatments.

MedlinePlus—Hair Diseases and Hair Loss <http://www.nlm.nih.gov/medlineplus/hairdiseasesandhairloss.html>

The MedlinePlus page on "Hair Diseases and Hair Loss" links to sites with basic information about causes, symptoms, and treatment of hair loss, plus has links to organizations, statistics, and more (see Figure 9.2).

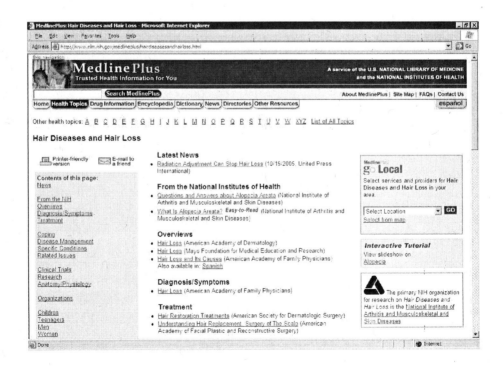

FIGURE 9.2. MedlinePlus—Hair Diseases and Hair Loss
<http://www.nlm.nih.gov/medlineplus/hairdiseasesandhairloss.html>

New Hair Institute
<http://www.newhair.com>

New Hair Institute (NHI) "is the pioneer of Follicular Unit Hair Transplantation and Follicular Unit Extraction." "NHI is a medical group of board certified physicians devoted solely to hair restoration." The NHI site contains basic information on hair loss and hair transplantation, a detailed description of follicular unit hair transplantation, and information about the new FOX procedure. The site promotes this medical group's services, which has several locations, and includes videos and a photo gallery, physician information, fees, and consultation/appointment services. The site now has a "Balding Blog" <BaldingBlog.com>.

NOAH—Hair Loss and Hair Disorders
<http://www.noah-health.org/en/skin/conditions/hair/index.html>

The NOAH page on hair loss includes links to subpages on hair loss anatomy, causes, surgical and nonsurgical treatment, and more. Within each page are links to peer-reviewed, quality Internet sources of information. NOAH pages are also available in Spanish.

Regrowth.com
<http://www.regrowth.com>

Despite this site's very commercial look, with ads placed throughout many of its pages, the content is easy to read and fairly neutral (nonsurgical treatments are preferred). The site was founded in 1996 and is still edited by Mr. John Ertel, who searched the Internet for his own hair loss problem and "was unable to find a comprehensive site that provided objective information." This site has information about hair loss and treatments (both surgical and nonsurgical), chat groups and forums, and much more; blogs are coming soon.

UpToDate Patient Information—Male Pattern Hair Loss (Androgenetic Alopecia)
<http://patients.uptodate.com/topic.asp?file=gen_hlth/2877

UpToDate is an evidence-based medicine product available to physicians. The patient information site has a select group of topics available for public use, including a page on male-pattern hair loss. The focus is on causes and diagnosis of hair loss and medical (drug) treatment, with a small section about surgery.

U.S. Food and Drug Administration—Hair Replacement: What Works, What Doesn't
<http://www.fda.gov/fdac/features/1997/397_hair.html>

This article by Larry Hanover originally appeared in the April 1997 FDA *Consumer* magazine. It covers everything from male-pattern baldness to health-related hair loss. The FDA's primary interest is medical treatment with products such as minoxidil, but hairpieces, surgery, and "mythical" treatments are all discussed.

NOTES

1. Hair Loss Learning Center. Available: <http://www.regrowhair.com>. Accessed: June 27, 2005.
2. Ibid.

Chapter 10

Cosmetic Dentistry

Cosmetic dentistry is an area that has gained prominence recently, partly due to its use in TV programs such as *Extreme Makeover* and *The Swan,* where dental work is done along with other cosmetic procedures. The American Academy of Cosmetic Dentistry, founded in 1984, offers accreditation and fellowship programs that provide "postgraduate and certification in cosmetic dentistry to both dentists and laboratory technicians." As new techniques and methods for improving the appearance of your teeth continue to be developed, this dental specialization seems poised to take off in popularity.

Treatments include whitening, bonding, dental implants, crowns, and veneers. Many procedures that are considered to be "cosmetic" can be done routinely in a dentist's office. Other procedures are more specialized, but your dentist will know who offers these cosmetic procedures in your area. If you are interested in improving the appearance of your teeth, it is important to become familiar with what cosmetic dental procedures are available and what might be appropriate for your needs.

Because each site includes descriptions of almost all cosmetic dental procedures, this chapter is not divided by procedure, but is organized alphabetically by the name of the site. Several specialties recognized by the American Dental Association may be involved with cosmetic procedures and are listed among these sites. Information about cosmetic dentistry applies equally to men and women.

Internet Guide to Cosmetic Surgery for Men
© 2006 by The Haworth Press, Inc. All rights reserved.
doi:10.1300/5854_11

COSMETIC DENTISTRY SITES

Academy of General Dentistry—Consumer Information
<http://www.agd.org/consumer>

The Academy of General Dentistry (AGD) is a membership organization of over 37,000 general dentists. They bill their Web site as the "'go to' dental resource for the general practitioner—and the organization for consumers to find reliable oral health information." From the "Consumer Information" page, you can link to "Oral Health Resources," "Find a Dentist," and a message board. Among the Oral Health Resources topics are: "Cosmetics," "Bleaching," "Crowns," "Implants," and "Veneers." Each of these pages then links to articles about the specific topic, for example, "Cosmetics" links to several articles, including "Improving Your Smile"; while "Veneers" links to articles such as "What are Porcelain Veneers?" "Dental Terms" links to brief definitions of dental terminology.

Aetna InteliHealth
<http://www.intelihealth.com>

InteliHealth is a quality consumer health site, with information primarily provided by the Harvard Medical School. The dental portion is provided by Columbia University School of Dental and Oral Surgery. Selecting "Dental Health" takes you to a commercial site, Simple Steps to Better Dental Health <http://www.simplestepsdental.com>, which is detailed later in this chapter.

American Academy of Cosmetic Dentistry
<http://www.aacd.com>

The American Academy of Cosmetic Dentistry (AACD) is "the world's largest organization of cosmetic dental professionals." Founded in 1984, the AACD "is dedicated to advancing the art and science of cosmetic dentistry." The AACD site (see Figure 10.1) is a great starting place for information about cosmetic dentistry. From the main page, in the "For the Pub-

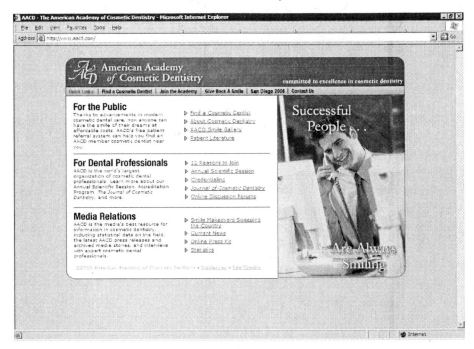

FIGURE 10.1. American Academy of Cosmetic Dentistry Home Page
<http://www.aacd.com>
Reprinted with permission of American Academy of Cosmetic Dentistry.

lic" section, you can link directly to "Find a Cosmetic Dentist," "About Cosmetic Dentistry," "AACD Smile Gallery," and "Patient Literature." Or, by clicking on "For the Public," you are taken to a page <http://www.aacd.com/public/default.aspx> that gives additional choices, including "AACD Extreme Makeover doctors" and a multimedia presentation. Additional links can be found by mousing over links on the top bar; you can find a glossary of terms, brief descriptions of procedures, and more extensive brochures on "The Art of Veneers," "The Art of Whitening," and "Your Smile Says it All!" This site has a cosmetic dentist finder. Also included is information for the media and for dental professionals.

American Academy of Periodontology
\<http://www.perio.org\>

The American Academy of Periodontology is one of nine specialty organizations recognized by the American Dental Association. This specialty deals with "the prevention, diagnosis and treatment of diseases affecting the gums and supporting structures of the teeth and in the placement and maintenance of dental implants." From the left-hand section, "For the Public," choose articles on "Dental Implants to Replace Teeth," "Plastic Surgery For Your Smile" (periodontal plastic procedures), and "Treatments to Save Your Teeth" (includes dental implants and cosmetic procedures). Or, from the menu bar near the top of the main page, mouse over "Public" and select from the pop-ups. Clicking "Public" from this menu bar takes you to the consumer page \<http://www.perio.org/consumer/index.html\>, which basically has the same information available from the main page. You can also locate a local periodontist via this site.

American Association of Orthodontists—Public Information
\<http://www.braces.org\>

Orthodontics, one of the nine specialties recognized by the American Dental Association, "is the branch of dentistry that specializes in the diagnosis, prevention and treatment of dental and facial irregularities." Orthodontists correct the bite, alignment, and spacing of teeth. From the main page, select "About Orthodontics" and then use links to connect to "Facts about Orthodontics," "Considering Orthodontic Treatment?" and more. Local orthodontists can be located via this site.

American College of Prosthodontists
\<http://www.prosthodontics.org\>

Prosthodontists are "specialists in the restoration and replacement of teeth." They specialize in restoring "function and esthetics to your smile" with procedures such as crowns, bridges, inlays, dentures, veneers, and dental implants. The American College of Prosthodontists is one of nine specialties recognized by the American Dental Association. From the main ACP page, select "Consumers/Patients" and then link to "Find a Prosthodontist." The site also includes "Improve Your Smile," "Consumer FAQ's," a photo gallery, and more.

American Dental Association
<http://www.ada.org>

The American Dental Association (ADA) "is the professional association of dentists committed to the public's health, ethics, science and professional advancement." On the ADA page, under "Your Oral Health," select "A-Z Topics." Topics include "Cosmetic Dentistry" <http://www.ada.org/public/topics/cosmetic.asp>, "Bridges," "Crowns," "Tooth Whitening Treatments," and "Veneers." Also available in "Your Oral Health" are "Frequently Asked Questions (FAQs)" and "Tips for Finding a Dentist." On the "A-Z Topics" page is a link to a very useful "Glossary of Terms" (left side of the page). This site has a dentist search feature, "Find an ADA Member Dentist."

Canadian Dental Association—Cosmetic Dentistry
<http://www.cda-adc.ca/en/oral_health>

Go directly to the URL or, from the CDA main page, select "Your Oral Health." Mouse over "Dental Procedures," and select from topics such as dental implants, bonding, and veneers. This site is also available in French.

Facial Plastic Surgery Network—Cosmetic Dentistry
<http://www.facialplasticsurgery.net/cosmetic_dentistry.htm>

This page can be reached directly via the URL, or go to the main page <http://www.facialplasticsurgery.net>, select "Facial Procedures," and then "Cosmetic Dental." This page is similar (orthodontics, tooth whitening, porcelain veneers and crowns, and gums) to **Yes They're Fake!**

iEnhance—Cosmetic Dentistry
<http://www.ienhance.com/speciality/dentistry.asp>

This page links to "Cosmetic Dentistry" (*sic*—speciality in URL), from which you can find a cosmetic dental specialist; go to the photo gallery, learn about cosmetic procedures, and ask questions of a cosmetic dentist. Or, you can go directly to the list of cosmetic procedures at <http://www.ienhance.com/procedures/procedure_list.asp?SpecialtyID=3>. The procedures list on this site is perhaps the most comprehensive of the cosmetic dentistry sites, and includes composite bonding, crowns, tooth whitening, porcelain veneers, cerinate veneers, dental implants, tooth contouring, and more. For each topic, the procedure is described, along with what to expect afterward, "ideal" candidates, risks, approximate costs, questions to ask your dentist, and more.

MedlinePlus—Cosmetic Dentistry
<http://www.nlm.nih.gov/medlineplus/cosmeticdentistry.html>

The MedlinePlus site links you to quality Web sites about cosmetic dentistry (see Figure 10.2). MedlinePlus is produced by the National Library of Medicine specifically for patients and health care consumers, and is always an excellent place to begin your search.

Simple Steps to Better Dental Health
<http://www.simplestepsdental.com>

You can find this site via Aetna InteliHealth (listed earlier in this chapter), or go directly to the Simple Steps Web site. This site is jointly sponsored by Aetna and Columbia University School of Dental and Oral Surgery. From this main page, select "Cosmetic Dentistry" (listed under "General Topics"), and then link to a variety of cosmetic dentistry topics— whitening, bonding, crown lengthening, veneers, recontouring, inlays, general information, and more. Transcripts are available from some of the chat sessions from this site. Also of interest from "General Topics" is "Orthodontics" and "Periodontics."

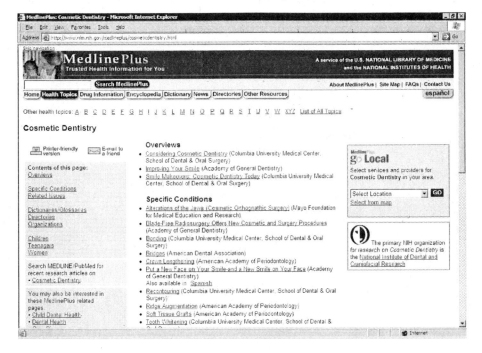

FIGURE 10.2. MedlinePlus—Cosmetic Dentistry
<http://www.nlm.nih.gov/medlineplus/cosmeticdentistry.html>

University of Iowa College of Dentistry—Cosmetic Dentistry
<http://www.dentistry.uiowa.edu/public/oral/
 cosmetic percent20dentistry.html>

This page from the College of Dentistry of the University of Iowa includes information on bonding, crowns, veneers, and tooth whitening.

WebMDHealth—Dental Health Center
<http://my.webmd.com/health_and_wellness/living_better/
 dental_health_center/default.htm>

WebMD is a reliable health information provider, and has fairly extensive information about cosmetic dentistry in general, and about specific procedures such as teeth whitening, veneers, crowns, restorations, bonding, recontouring, and more. This information is provided in collaboration with the Cleveland Clinic. You can go directly to the "Dental Health Center" using the URL and then select "Cosmetic Dentistry" and then specific procedures; or, go to <http://www.webmd.com>, search for "Cosmetic Dentistry," choose the "Dental Health Center," and then "Cosmetic Dentistry." This site displays the HONcode.

Yes They're Fake!—Cosmetic Dentistry
<http://www.yestheyrefake.net/cosmetic_dental.html>

This candid site was created by a patient who has undergone cosmetic surgery and includes everything from over-the-counter whitening products (e.g., Crest Whitestrips), to professional whitening systems and laser whitening. Other cosmetic dentistry topics listed include orthodontics, porcelain crowns and veneers, bonding, and gum surgery. Average prices for dental procedures are given. You can access this information by going directly to the URL, or go to the main page <http://www.yestheyrefake.net>, select "Facial Procedures," and then "Cosmetic Dentistry."

Chapter 11

Cosmetic Surgery and Ethnicity

In recent years, cosmetic surgery has increased among minorities in the United States. According to the American Society for Aesthetic Plastic Surgery, in 2001, minorities accounted for 17 percent of all cosmetic surgery procedures. The breakdown by ethnicity was: 7 percent Hispanic, 5 percent African American, 4 percent Asian, and 1 percent other non-Caucasian.[1] By 2004, the number of procedures in minorities had increased to 20 percent of all surgeries, with a breakdown of 8.5 percent in Hispanics, 6.2 percent in African Americans, 4.6 percent in Asians, and 1.1 percent in other non-Caucasians.[2] Statistics from the American Society of Plastic Surgeons indicate that in 2004, Hispanics accounted for 6 percent (552,638) of procedures, African Americans for 5 percent (460,531 procedures), Asian Americans for 3 percent (276,319 procedures), and other minorities for 1 percent (92,106).[3]

Although many procedures remain the same across all ethnicities, some are greatly influenced by the patient's ethnic/racial type. The increase in numbers of minorities electing cosmetic surgery has created the need for surgeons to understand the differences that are caused by racial background. With an "increased awareness about ethnic concerns and new procedures that cater to the inherent differences" in skin color, facial features, and body structure, blacks and other minorities have found that they can consider cosmetic surgery without "cutting off a piece of their heritage."[4]

Many physicians now specialize in cosmetic surgery for specific minorities. In fact, the Internet has many sites put up by doctor's offices that specialize in cosmetic surgery for minorities. This chapter offers a group of sites to get you started in your search for ethnicity in cosmetic surgery. Sites are listed alphabetically, without regard for race/ethnicity, or cosmetic procedure. Hopefully, more information concerning ethnic minorities will appear on the Web sites of the major cosmetic surgery organizations in the near

Internet Guide to Cosmetic Surgery for Men
© 2006 by The Haworth Press, Inc. All rights reserved.
doi:10.1300/5854_12

future. Should you wish to check out specific practice sites, search terms for you to consider using in a search engine include: "cosmetic surgery" with: ethnic," "ethnicity," "minorities," "African American," "Hispanic," or "Asian, for example, "African American cosmetic surgery."

ETHNIC COSMETIC SURGERY SITES

American Academy of Facial Plastic and Reconstructive Surgeons
<http://www.aafprs.org>

The AAFPRS has several articles in their online newsletter, *Facial Plastic Surgery Today,* of interest to minorities. These are: "Ethnic Differences and Facial Plastic Surgery," "Recent Survey Reveals Increase in Cosmetic Surgery," and "Your Eyes Tell it All; Ethnicity Plays a Part—Explore Your Surgical Options." These articles could not be accessed directly using a URL; to locate them, use the site search for terms such as "ethnic" "Asian," etc.

American Society of Plastic Surgeons
<http://www.plasticsurgery.org>

The ASPS, in addition to providing annual statistics that include an ethnic breakdown, has issued several press releases about cosmetic surgery in minorities: "African-Americans Maintain Ethnic Identify with Nose Reshaping" (April 7, 2003), "Asian Plastic Surgery Patients Benefit from New Techniques in Cosmetic Surgery" (May 31, 2002), "Half-Million Cosmetic Plastic Surgery Procedures For Hispanics in 2004—Up 49 percent From 2000" (March 16, 2005), and "Innovations in Scar Management Offer Encouraging News for African American Plastic Surgery Patients" (January 31, 2003). Press releases can be reached by selecting "News Room" from the main page and then "Press Releases." They are in reverse order by date.

Bermant Plastic and Cosmetic Surgery
<http://www.plasticsurgery4u.com>

This site is provided by Dr. Michael Bermant, a board-certified physician in plastic surgery, who practices near Richmond, VA. A wealth of examples of cosmetic surgery on minorities/ethnic groups is available on this site. The easiest approach is to use "Search this Site" for appropriate words such as "ethnic," "African," and "Asian." You can be quite specific, e.g., "ethnic nose" would locate a page called "Ethnic Black Rhinoplasty in a Male Patient." Hundreds of examples of surgeries on ethnic patients are available.

CosmeticSurgery.com—Ethnic Considerations in Plastic Surgery
<http://www.cosmeticsurgery.com/articles/archive/an~134/>

This news feature on ethnic aspects of cosmetic surgery focuses on skin differences between persons of different backgrounds. A chart compares skin type, ethnic background, sun history, aging, and challenges.

eMedicine
<http://www.emedicine.com>

A search of eMedicine finds a number of articles about cosmetic surgery in minorities/ethnic patients. Articles are written by physicians and may be a bit technical. Use the "Search" feature, type in phrases such as "ethnic cosmetic surgery" to locate articles such as:

> "Rhinoplasty, Asian"
> <http://www.emedicine.com/plastic/topic474.htm>
> "Rhinoplasty, Multiracial"
> <http://www.emedicine.com/ent/topic113.htm>
> "Craniofacial, Asian Malar and Mandibular Surgery"
> <http://www.emedicine.com/plastic/topic427.htm>
> "Facial Plastic Surgery in Asian Patients"
> <http://www.emedicine.com/ent/topic680.htm>

Information is free, but you must register to use eMedicine.

iEnhance—Asian Eyes—Blepharoplasty
<http://www.ienhance.com/procedure/default.asp>

Link directly to the "Procedures" page and select either "Plastic Surgery" or "Facial Plastic Surgery," then under "Head/Face" select "Asian Eyes—Blepharoplasty." The page describes the "single eyelid" that is common in the Asian population and the surgery that can create a double upper eyelid. The page includes basic information about the surgical procedure, risks, postsurgical recovery, and questions to ask your doctor.

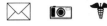

NOTES

1. American Society for Aesthetic Plastic Surgery. "Cosmetic Procedures Increase To Nearly 8.5 Million, Says American Society For Aesthetic Plastic Surgery." (Press release, February 20, 2002). Available: <http://surgery.org/press/0202-increase.php>. Accessed: October 19, 2005.

2. American Society for Aesthetic Plastic Surgery. "11.9 Million Cosmetic Procedures in 2004." (Press release, February 17, 2005). Available: <http://www.surgery.org/press/news-print.php?iid=395>. Accessed: March 8, 2005.

3. American Society of Plastic Surgeons. "2004 Cosmetic Demographics, Patient Ethnicity, Body Contouring After Massive Weight Loss." Available: <http://www.plastic surgery.org/public_education/2004Statistics.cfm>. Accessed: October 19, 2005.

4. Barrow, Karen. "Saving Face: Ethnic Concerns in Plastic Surgery." ABC News, June 1, 2005. Available: <http://absnews.go.com/Health/cosmetic/story?id=809747>. Accessed: October 18, 2005.

Chapter 12

International Cosmetic Surgery Associations

Information in the previous chapters has been primarily from U.S. Web sites. Readers from outside the United States will find much valuable information from these U.S. sites. However, excellent non-U.S. sources are also available that will be relevant and useful to both U.S. and non-U.S. readers who are considering cosmetic surgery. Cosmetic surgery is just becoming more commonplace in the United States but has been considered "routine" in many other countries for some time now. Worldwide, many people take vacations that incorporate cosmetic surgery and recovery time.

This selected list consists of non-U.S. professional associations specializing in cosmetic surgery and plastic surgery, and related medical specialties. It is not intended to be comprehensive and is weighted heavily toward English-speaking countries. Also, selected sites must have information intended for health consumers or patients in order to be included here. Sites intended primarily for physicians are excluded.

Information provided by a professional association or society in your country (or the country in which you plan on having your surgery) is the best place to start. The Web site will usually give overview information for many procedures, indicate standards for member physicians, and provide a list of accredited cosmetic or plastic surgeons (some with links to the surgeons' Web sites). Web sites for international (including multinational) associations/organizations are listed first, followed by associations from specific countries. This list is only a sample of cosmetic surgery organizations worldwide.

Tip: If you find that a URL does not work, search for the main words of the association in your search browser or on a search engine such as Google.

Internet Guide to Cosmetic Surgery for Men
© 2006 by The Haworth Press, Inc. All rights reserved.
doi:10.1300/5854_13

INTERNATIONAL/MULTINATIONAL ASSOCIATIONS

European Academy of Facial Plastic Surgery
\<http://www.eafps.com\>

Select "Patient Information" to get to information about procedures and a membership list searchable by name or country. The procedure information (eight procedures) is reprinted with permission from the American Academy of Facial Plastic and Reconstructive Surgery.

International Confederation for Plastic, Reconstructive
and Aesthetic Surgery (IPRAS)—World Plastic Surgery
\<http://www.ipras.org\>

IPRAS promotes plastic surgery, both clinically and scientifically, worldwide. "Public Info" is limited to locating physicians in member countries.

International Society of Aesthetic Plastic Surgery
\<http://www.isaps.org/\>

This site is intended for the public to "provide it with information regarding organization and practice of Aesthetic Plastic Surgery all around the world." The site provides general information along with a list of qualified plastic surgeons and their home country.

PLink: The Plastic Surgery Links Collection
\<http://www.nvpc.nl/plink\>

This site, created by the Netherlands Society for Plastic Surgery, is a searchable database of links to sites on the Internet that deal with plastic surgery. Links are to doctors' sites, patients' sites, subjects, and more, all related to plastic surgery. This is a great site to locate plastic surgery organizations by country.

COSMETIC SURGERY ASSOCIATIONS BY COUNTRY

Argentina

Sociedad Argentina de Cirugía Plástica, Estética y Reparadora (SACPER)
<http://www.cirplastica.org.ar/>

This site is in Spanish. Select "Procedimientos" for a patient information about specific procedures; includes membership information (locate a physician).

Sociedad de Cirugía Plástica de Buenos Aires
<http://www.scpba.intramed.net.ar/>

This site is in Spanish, with some English sections. Over twenty procedures are listed in the Spanish version. "Miembros" is an alphabetical list of members.

Australia

Australian Society of Plastic Surgeons
<http://www.plasticsurgery.org.au>

This site is the location for Australians to begin their search for plastic surgery information. Articles on a variety of procedures are available along with a database of society members searchable by location, name, and procedures. Also included are links to other associations and a list of FAQs.

Canada

Canadian Academy of Facial Plastic and Reconstructive Surgery
<http://www.facialcosmeticsurgery.org>

This site has a physician locator and information on surgical procedures (e.g., browlift, rhinoplasty, otoplasty, hair restoration), nonsurgical cosmetic procedures (e.g., Botox, microdermabrasion, fat transfer), and a photo gallery, in addition to information for member physicians.

Canadian Laser Aesthetic Surgery Society (CLASS)
<http://www.class.ca/>

Locate a member, plus information on cosmetic procedures. This site is in English and French.

Canadian Society for Aesthetic (Cosmetic) Plastic Surgery
<http://www.csaps.ca>

The CSAPS site includes information about surgical procedures, along with a Find a Surgeon feature. This site can also be reached from the **Canadian Society of Plastic Surgeons <http://www.plasticsurgery.ca>** by selecting "Aesthetic Plastic Surgery Site." Information is available in English and French.

Canadian Society of Plastic Surgeons
<http://www.plasticsurgery.ca/>

This professional society seeks to advance the practice of cosmetic surgery. Enter the site by selecting English or French. Select "Surgeon Referral" to locate a plastic surgeon, "Procedures" for information about the most common plastic surgery procedures, or "Aesthetic Plastic Surgery Site" to take you to <http://www.csaps.ca> for further public information. This site is in English and French.

Cosmetic Surgery Canada
<http://cosmeticsurgerycanada.com/>

This is a commercial site that provides a surgeon search and referral service.

England

See Great Britain.

France

Société Francaise de Chirurgie Plastique Reconstructrice et Esthétique (SFCPRE)
\<http://www.plasticiens.org\>

In French. For a description of procedures, select "Interventions." Has FAQs.

Société Francaise des Chirurgiens Esthétiques Plasticiens (French Society of Aesthetic Plastic Surgery)
\<http://www.sofcep.org/\>

In French. An English front-end page can be found at \<http://www. sofcep.org/uk/index.htm\>.

Germany

Vereinigung der Deutschen Aesthetisch-Plastischen Chirurgen
\<http://www.vdaepc.de/\>

In German. Select "Patienteninformationen."

Vereinigung der Deutschen Plastischen Chirurgen
\<http://www.vdpc.de\>

In German.

Great Britain

British Association of Aesthetic Plastic Surgeons (BAAPS)
\<http://www.baaps.org.uk\>

BAAPS was founded to advance "education in, and the practice of, aesthetic plastic surgery for public interest." This site includes a "Find a Surgeon" feature along with information about cosmetic procedures. Selecting "About Plastic Surgery" will locate qualifications and reasons why to select a BAAPS member surgeon, descriptions of many plastic surgery procedures, and FAQs.

British Association of Plastic Surgeons
<http://www.baps.co.uk/>

"The Association is the professional representative body for plastic and reconstructive surgeons in the United Kingdom," and is therefore the recommended location for readers located in Great Britain to begin their search for information. The site contains information on procedures and members.

British Society for Surgery of the Hand
<http://www.bssh.ac.uk>

Select "Resources," and then select from Patient Leaflets, Publications, Links, Members, and Support Groups.

Italy

Società Italiana di Chirurgia Plastica Ricostruttiva ed Estetica
<http://www.sicpre.org>

In Italian. Select "Interventi estetici" for descriptions of cosmetic procedures.

Mexico

Asociación Mexicana de Cirugía Plástica, Estética y Reconstructiva
<http://www.cirugiaplastica.org.mx/>

In Spanish. An English version is available at <http://www.plastic surgery.org.mx>. The site includes information about selecting a qualified surgeon, and membership requirements; this site is primarily a directory of members.

Netherlands

Nederlandse Vereniging voor Plastische Chirurgie
<http://www.nvpc.nl/nvpc/index.htm>

This site, in Dutch, gives information on plastic surgery for both patients and doctors. This site is the home of PLink (the Plastic Surgery

Links Collection), an aggregator of plastic surgery information. The PLink site is in English.

South Africa

Association of Plastic and Reconstructive Surgeons of Southern Africa
<http://www.plasticsurgeons.co.za>

Includes information on finding a plastic surgeon in South Africa along with "Overseas Information" for patients who are coming to South Africa for surgery. Brief patient information on procedures is available in "Questions & Answers" and "Articles of Interest," but this site relies on links to other organizations to provide more detailed information about plastic surgery procedures.

Spain

Sociedad Española de Cirugia Plástica, Reparadora y Estética (SECPRE)
<http://www.secpre.org>

In Spanish. Select "Información para pacientes."

Switzerland

Societe Suisse de Chirurgie Plastique, Reconstructive et Esthetique
<http://www.plastic-surgery.ch>

This site presents basic information for residents of Switzerland, including site location of surgeons and health insurance. Links to other organizations worldwide are provided for descriptions of surgical procedures. Select German or French to enter this site.

Turkey

Türk Plastik Rekonstrüktif ve Estetik Cerrahi Derneği (Turkish Society of Plastic, Reconstructive and Aesthetic Surgeons) <http://www.tpcd.org.tr/>

In Turkish.

United Kingdom

See Great Britain.

Index

Abdominal liposculpture, 54
Abdominal liposuction. *See* Abdominal
    liposculpture
Abdominoplasty. *See* Tummy tuck
    (Abdominoplasty)
ABMS. *See* American Board of Medical
    Specialists
About.com, Men's Health – cosmetic
    surgery and men, 49
Academy of General Dentistry, 176
Aetna InteliHealth, 176
AgingSkinNet, skin (general), 121-122
All About Cheek Augmentation, 90
All About Chin Augmentation, 92
All About Jaw Augmentation, 110
All About Lip Augmentation, 112
AlltheWeb, 19
Alta Vista, 19
American Academy of Cosmetic
    Dentistry, 176-177
American Academy of Cosmetic Surgery
  abdominoplasty (tummy tuck), 69
  buttock implants, 57
  calf implants, 58
  collagen, 138
  core site, 36-37
  fat injections, 138
  gynecomastia, 74
  Hyalaform, 140
  laser surfacing, 143
  liposuction, 60
  Restylane, 140
  sclerotherapy (veins), 152
  thermage, 158
  thighlift, 68
  upper arm lift, 55

American Academy of Dermatology
  botulinum toxin, 125
  cellulite, 129
  chemical peeling, 130
  core site, 37-38
  dermabrasion, 132
  facial skin rejuvenation, 159
  hair restoration, 163
  laser resurfacing, 143
  scars, 149
  skin (general), 122-123
  soft tissue fillers, 135
  spider veins, varicose vein therapy, 152
  tattoos, body piercings, and other skin
    adornments, 147
  tumescent liposuction, 60
American Academy of Facial Plastic and
    Reconstructive Surgery
  blepharoplasty, 97
  Botox injections, 125
  core site, 38-39
  ethnicity, 194
  face, head, and neck surgery, 85-86
  facial scar treatment, 150
  forehead and brow lift surgery, 107
  hair replacement surgery, 164
  mentoplasty surgery, 92, 93
  otoplasty surgery, 94-95
  rhinoplasty surgery, 115
  rhytidectomy, 100
  skin resurfacing, 155
  wrinkle treatment, 159
American Academy of Otolaryngology –
    Head and Neck Surgery
  ear surgery, 95
  nose surgery, 116

Internet Guide to Cosmetic Surgery for Men
© 2006 by The Haworth Press, Inc. All rights reserved.
doi:10.1300/5854_14

American Academy of Periodontology, 178
American Association of Orthodontists, 178
American Board of Cosmetic Surgery, 31
American Board of Dermatology, 29-30
American Board of Facial Plastic and Reconstructive Surgery, 32
American Board of Hair Restoration Surgery, 165
American Board of Medical Specialists, 28-31
American Board of Ophthalmology, 30
American Board of Oral and Maxillofacial Surgery, 31
American Board of Otolaryngology, 30
American Board of Plastic Surgery, 29
American Board of Surgery, 30-31
American College of Prosthodontists, 178-179
American Dental Association, 179
American Hair Loss Council, 165
American Skincare and Cellulite Expert Association, 129
American Society for Aesthetic Plastic Surgery
    botulinum toxin injections, 125
    chemical skin peel (light and deep), 130
    collagen injections, 138
    core site, 39-41
    eyelid surgery, 98
    facelift, 100
    facial implants, 104
    fat injection, 138
    forehead lift, 107
    gynecomastia, 75
    hair transplantation, 165
    injectables, 136
    laser hair removal, 141
    lip augmentation, 112
    liposuction, 61
    male breast reduction (gynecomastia), 75
    men: penile augmentation by fat injection, 82
    microdermabrasion, 146
American Society for Aesthetic Plastic Surgery *(continued)*
    micropigmentation, 148
    nose reshaping, 116
    sclerotherapy, 153
    skin resurfacing, 155
    statistics, 9
    tummy tuck, 69
American Society for Dermatologic Surgery
    aging eyelids, 98
    botulinum toxin treatments, 126
    chemical peeling, 131
    core site, 41-42
    dermabrasion, 133
    hair restoration treatments, 166
    laser hair removal, 142
    laser resurfacing, 143
    liposuction surgery, 61, 62
    microlipoinjection (or fat transfer), 139
    Restylane, 140
    skin (general), 123
    spider and varicose veins, 153-154
    tattoo removal, 156
American Society of Ophthalmic Plastic and Reconstructive Surgery, core site, 42
American Society of Plastic Surgeons
    abdominoplasty (tummy tuck), 69
    blepharoplasty (eyelids), 98
    brachioplasty, 56
    browlift (forehead lift), 107-108
    chemical peel, 131
    chin surgery, 92
    core site, 42-44
    dermabrasion, 133, 134
    ethnicity, 184
    facial implants (chin, cheeks, and jaw surgery), 105
    facial rejuvenation (Botox), 126
    gynecomastia, 75, 76
    hair replacement, 166
    injectable fillers, 136, 137
    laser skin resurfacing, 144
    lipoplasty (liposuction), 61-62
    male breast reduction, 75, 76

American Society of Plastic Surgeons
  (continued)
  men's plastic surgery, 49, 50
  microdermabrasion, 146
  otoplasty (ear surgery), 96
  permanent eyeliner, 148
  rhinoplasty (surgery of the nose),
    116-117
  rhytidectomy (facelift), 101
  scar revision, 151
  sclerotherapy (spider veins), 154
  skin management (surface-repair
    treatments), 159
  skin resurfacing, 155
  statistics, 8-9
Arm lift, 54-56
Arm liposuction. *See* Arm lift
Ask Jeeves, 19
Ask NOAH About, 21-22, 36
  hair loss and hair disorders, 173
Asociación Mexicana de Cirugía Plástica,
    Esthética y Reconstructiva, 192
Association of Plastic and Reconstructive
    Surgeons of Southern Africa, 193
Australian Society of Plastic Surgeons,
    189

Baby boomers, 8
Belt lipectomy. *See* Lower body lift
Bermant Plastic and Cosmetic Surgery
  blepharoplasty (eyelid cosmetic
    surgery), 99
  body contouring, 53-54
  brow lift (forehead lift), 108
  ethnicity, 184-185
  eyelid sculpture, 99
  facelift surgery, 102
  gynecomastia, 75
  male plastic surgery, 49
  nasal sculpture, 117
  otoplasty, 96
Blepharoplasty. *See* Eyelid surgery
    (Blepharoplasty)
Board certification, 27-33

Body contouring, 53-71
BodyImplants.com, pec implants (pectoral
    augmentation), 79
Body lift. *See* Lower body lift
Botox. *See* Botulinum Toxin (Botox)
    injections
Botulinum Toxin (Botox) injections,
    124-128
Brachioplasty. *See* Arm lift
Breast reduction, male. *See* Gynecomastia
British Association of Aesthetic Plastic
    Surgeons (BAAPS), 191
British Association of Plastic Surgeons,
    192
British Society for Surgery of the Hand,
    192
Brow lift. *See* Forehead lift (brow lift)
Browsers, 18
Buccal fat pad removal, 89-90
Buttock augmentation/implant, 57
Buttock implant. *See* Buttock
    augmentation/implant
Buttock lift/liposculpture/liposuction,
    57-58
Buttock liposuction. *See* Buttock
    lift/liposculpture/liposuction

Calf augmentation/implants, 58-59
Canadian Academy of Facial Plastic and
    Reconstructive Surgery, 189
Canadian Dental Association, 179
Canadian Laser Aesthetic Surgery Society
    (CLASS), 190
Canadian Society for Aesthetic (Cosmetic)
    Plastic Surgery, 190
Canadian Society of Plastic Surgeons, 190
Cellulite treatment, 128-129
Central body lift. *See* Lower body lift
Cheek augmentation. *See* Cheek implants
    (Augmentation)
Cheek implants (Augmentation), 90-91
Cheek reduction. *See* Buccal fat pad
    removal
Chemical peels, 130-132

Chin augmentation (Mentoplasty), 91-94
Collagen injections, 137-138
Columbia University Department of
      Surgery, upper arm lift, 56
Cosmetic dentistry, 175-182
Cosmetic surgeons
      credentials/board certification, 27-33
      locating online, 25-27, 33-34
      selecting, 25-27, 33-34
Cosmetic surgery
      baby boomers, 8
      basic/core sites for men, 35-52
      and celebrities, 7
      cost, 10
      ethnicity, 183-186
      statistics, 8-9
      trends, 6
Cosmetic Surgery Canada, 190
Cosmetic Surgery FYI, core site, 44-45
CosmeticSurgery.com, ethnic
      considerations, 185
Credentialing, 25-34

Dentistry, cosmetic. *See* Cosmetic
      dentistry
Dermabrasion, 132-134
Dogpile, 19, 20

Ear surgery (Otoplasty), 94-97
eMedicine
      body contouring, buttocks surgery, 58
      body contouring, flankoplasty and
            thigh lift, 67
      ethnicity, 185
      gynecomastia, 75-76
      hair replacement surgery, 166-167
      liposuction, upper arms, 56
Endermologie. *See* Cellulite treatment
Ethnicity, 183-186
European Academy of Facial Plastic
      Surgery, 188
Evaluating information, 15-17
Eyelid surgery (Blepharoplasty), 97-100

Face, head, and neck surgery, 85-119
Facelift (Rhytidectomy), 100-103
Facelift FYI, 102
Facial implants, 103-105
Facial liposuction, 105-106
Facial Plastic Surgery Network
      blepharoplasty (eyelid tuck surgery), 99
      buccal fat pad extraction, 89
      chemical peels, 131
      core site, 45-46
      cosmetic dentistry, 179
      dermabrasion, 133
      face, head, and neck surgery, 87
      face lift, 102
      facial and neck liposuction, 105-106
      facial fat grafting (fat transfer), 139
      forehead and brow lift surgery, 109
      injectables, 136
      jaw augmentation and jaw implants,
            110, 111
      laser resurfacing and laser treatments,
            144
      lip reduction, 113
      microdermabrasion, 147
      micropigmentation (permanent
            makeup), 148
      neck lift (platysmaplasty), 114
      otoplasty, 96
      scar revision and keloid prevention, 151
      skin (general), 123
      tattoo removal, 156, 157
Fat injections, 138-139
FDA. *See* U.S. FDA
Flankoplasty. *See* Lower body lift
Forehead lift (Brow lift), 107-109

Google, 17, 19, 20
Gynecomastia (Male breast reduction),
      73-77

Hair Loss Learning Center, 167
Hair Loss Patient Guide, 167-168
Hair Loss Research, 168
Hair Loss Scams!, 168

Hair Loss Specialists, 168-169
Hair replacement. *See* Hair transplantation
Hair Transplant Adviser, 169
Hair Transplant Medical, 169-170
Hair Transplant Network, 170
Hair transplantation, 161-174
Head surgery. *See* Face, head, and neck surgery
Health on the Net (HON), 16
HotBot, 19
Hyaluronic acid injections, 140-141
Hypertext markup language, 14
Hypertext transfer protocol, 14

iEnhance
  abdominal liposculpture, 54, 55
  abdominoplasty (tummy tuck), 69
  arm liposuction, 56
  Asian eyes – blepharoplasty, 185-186
  Botox® Cosmetic, 126
  buttock liposculpture/liposuction, 58
  calf implants, 59
  cheek augmentation/implants, 90-91
  chemical peel, 131
  chin augmentation/implants, 92-93
  core site, 46-47
  cosmetic dentistry, 180
  dermabrasion, 133
  ear surgery (otoplasty), 96-97
  eyelid surgery (blepharoplasty), 99
  face lift, 102-103
  facial plastic surgery, 87, 88, 124
  fat injections, 139
  forehead lift, 109
  gynecomastia (male breast), 76-77
  laser hair removal, 142
  laser skin resurfacing, 144
  laser spider vein treatment, 145
  lip augmentation, 112
  liposculpture/liposuction, 62-63
  male breast reduction, 76-77
  male pectoral implants, 79
  neck liposuction, 114
  nose surgery (rhinoplasty), 118

iEnhance *(continued)*
  permanent cosmetics, 148
  Restylane, 140
  scar revision/scar repair, 151
  skin (general), 124
  skin injection treatments, 136-137
  spider vein treatment (sclerotherapy), 154
  tattoo removal, 156
  thigh liposculpture, 68
InfoPlasticSurgery.com, pectoral augmentation, 79
Injectable fillers, 135-141
Institute of Cosmetic Surgery, male cosmetic surgery, 50
InteliHealth. *See* Aetna InteliHealth
International Alliance of Hair Restoration Surgeons, 170
International Confederation for Plastic, Reconstructive and Aesthetic Surgery (IPRAS), 188
International cosmetic surgery associations, 187-194
International Hair Transplant Institute, 171
International Society of Aesthetic Plastic Surgery, 188
International Society of Hair Restoration Surgery, 171
Internet, 13-24
  addresses, 14
  basic searching, 17
  basic/core sites on cosmetic surgery, 35-52
  browsers, 18
  megasites, 21-24
  search engine directories, 18-21
Internet Explorer, 17-18
Ixquick Metasearch, 19

Jaw augmentation, 109-111

Laser hair removal, 141-145
Laser skin resurfacing, 142-145. *See also* Chemical peels; Dermabrasion

Laser treatment of spider veins, 145-146
Lip augmentation, 111-113
Lip reduction, 113
Lipoinfo.com, 63
Liposuction, 59-66
Liposuction 4 You, 63-64
Liposuction Consumer Guide, 64-65
LiposuctionFYI.com, 65
LookSmart, 19
Lower body lift, 67

Mamma, 17, 19
Mastopexy. *See* Breast lift (Mastopexy)
MayoClinic.com
    facelifts, 103
    laser hair removal, 142
    laser resurfacing, 145
    liposuction, 65
    penis-enlargement scams, 82
Medem
    core site, 47-48
    male pattern baldness, 171-172
MedlinePlus, 22-24, 36
    Botox, 127
    cosmetic dentistry, 180-181
    hair diseases and hair loss, 172
Megasites, 21-24
Mentoplasty. *See* Chin augmentation
        (Mentoplasty)
MetaCrawler, 19
Microdermabrasion, 146-147
Micropigmentation (Permanent makeup),
        147-149

National Library of Medicine, 22-23
Neck lift/Neck liposuction, 114-115
Neck liposuction. *See* Neck lift/Neck
        Liposuction
Neck surgery. *See* Face, head, and neck
        surgery
Nederlandse Vereniging voor Plastische
        Chirurgie, 192
Netscape, 17-18

New Hair Institute, 173
New York Online Access to Health. *See*
        Ask NOAH About
New York Phallo, 82-83
NOAH. *See* Ask NOAH About
Nose surgery (Rhinoplasty), 115-119

Otoplasty. *See* Ear surgery (Otoplasty)

Pec Implants.com
    gynecomastia, 77
    pec implants (pectoral augmentation),
        80
Pectoral (male chest) augmentation/
        implants, 77-80
Penis enlargement/implants (Phalloplasty),
        80-84
Penis-Enlargement.com, 83
Permanent cosmetics. *See*
        Micropigmentation (Permanent
        makeup)
Permanent makeup. *See*
        Micropigmentation (Permanent
        makeup)
Phalloplasty. *See* Penis enlargement/
        implants (Phalloplasty)
Plastic surgery, 6
Plastic Surgery 4 Men, 50-51
PLink; The Plastic Surgery Links
        Collection, 188
Professional membership organizations,
        32-33

Regrowth.com, 173
Rhinoplasty. *See* Nose surgery
        (Rhinoplasty)
Rhinoplasty 4 You, 118
Rhinoplasty FYI, 118
Rhytidectomy. *See* Facelift
        (Rhytidectomy)

Scar revision. *See* Scars/scar revision
Scars/scar revision, 149-152
Sclerotherapy, 152-154
Search engine directories, 18-21
Search engines, 19
Simple Steps to Better Dental Health, 180
Skin management. *See* Botulinum toxin
  (Botox) injections; Chemical
  peels; Dermabrasion; Injectable
  fillers; Laser skin resurfacing;
  Skin resurfacing; Wrinkle
  treatment
Skin resurfacing, 154-155
Skin surgery, 121-160
Sociedad Argentina de Cirugía Plástica,
  Estética y Reparadora
  (SACPER), 189
Sociedad de Cirugía Plástica de Buenos
  Aires, 189
Sociedad Española de Cirugia Plástica,
  Reparadora y Estética
  (SECPRE), 193
Società Italiana di Chirurgia Plastica
  Riconstructtiva ed Esthetica, 192
Société Francaise de Chirurgie Plastique
  Reconstructice et Esthétique
  (SFCPRE), 191
Société Francaise des Chirurgiens
  Esthétiques Plasticiens (French
  Society of Aesthetic Plastic
  Surgery), 191
Société Suisse de Chirurgie Plastique,
  Reconstructive et Esthétique, 193
Soft tissue fillers. *See* Injectable fillers
Spider veins. *See* Laser treatment of spider
  veins; Sclerotherapy

Tattoo removal, 156-157. *See also*
  Dermabrasion and Laser skin
  resurfacing
Teoma, 19
Thermage, 158
Thigh lift. *See* Thigh liposuction
  (Thighplasty)/Thigh lift

Thigh liposuction (Thighplasty)/Thigh lift,
  67-68
Thighplasty. *See* Thigh liposuction
  (Thighplasty)/Thigh lift
Tuck That Tummy!, 70
Tummy tuck (Abdominoplasty), 68-70
Tummy Tuck Resource, 70
Türk Plastik Rekonstrüktif ve Estetik
  Cerrahi Derneği (Turkish Society
  of Plastic, Reconstructive and
  Aesthetic Surgeons), 194

Uniform resource locator (URL), 14
University of Iowa College of Dentistry,
  cosmetic dentistry, 181
University of Iowa Health Care, belt
  lipectomy, 67
Upper arm lift. *See* Arm lift
  (Brachioplasty); Arm
  liposuction; Upper arm lift
UpToDate Patient Information, male
  pattern hair loss (androgenetic
  alopecia), 174
URAC. *See* Utilization Review Accreditation
  Commission (URAC)
URL. *See* Uniform resource locator (URL)
UrologyHealth.org, 83
U.S. Food and Drug Administration
  Botox cosmetic, 127-128
  hair restoration, 174
U.S. Food and Drug Administration. Center
  for Devices and Radiological
  Health
  Hyalaform, 141
  liposuction information, 65-66
  Restylane, 141
Utilization Review Accreditation
  Commission (URAC), 16

Vereinigung der Deutschen Aesthetisch-
  Plastischen Chirurgen, 191
Vereinigung der Deutschen Plastischen
  Chirurgen, 191
Vivisimo, 19, 20

Web site evaluation, 15-17
WebMDHealth, dental health center,
      181-182
World Wide Web, 14
Wrinkle treatment, 158-160. *See also*
      Botulinum toxin (Botox)
      injections; Chemical peels;
      Dermabrasion; Injectable fillers;
      Laser skin resurfacing

Yahoo!, 17, 19, 21
Yes They're Fake!
   abdominoplasty, 70
   blepharoplasty, 99-100
   body enhancement, 54
   Botox, 128
   brow or forehead lift, 109
   buccal fat pad removal, 90
   buttock augmentation, 57
   calf augmentation, 59
   cellulite treatment, 129
   cheek augmentation, 91
   chemical peels, 132
   chin augmentation, 93-94
   core site, 48

Yes They're Fake! *(continued)*
   cosmetic dentistry, 182
   dermabrasion, 134
   face, head, and neck (general), 87
   face lift, 103
   facial enhancement surgery, 87, 124
   facial implants, 105
   facial liposuction, 106
   fat grafting, 139
   gynecomastia, 77, 78
   jaw augmentation, 110
   laser treatments, 145
   lip augmentation, 113
   lip reduction, 113
   liposuction, 66
   microdermabrasion, 147
   micropigmentation, 149
   neck lift, 115
   otoplasty, 97
   pectoral implants, 80
   phalloplasty, 84
   rhinoplasty, 118-119
   scar revision, 151-152
   skin (general), 124
   tattoo removal, 157
   Thermacool thermaplasty, 158
   wrinkles, 160